Thank you!

Elwin George MD

BIG
MEDICINE:
THE COST OF CORPORATE CONTROL AND HOW DOCTORS AND PATIENTS WORKING TOGETHER CAN REBUILD A BETTER SYSTEM

By Elaina George, MD

Edited by Dave Racer, MLitt

Alethos Press – St Paul, MN

i

Alethos Press
1535 Barclay St, Ste B-1
St Paul MN 55106
alethospress@comcast.net

ISBN: 978-0-9849552-0-6

Big Medicine: The Cost of Corporate Control and How Doctors and Patients Working Together Can Rebuild a Better System

Author: Elaina George, MD

Edited by Dave Racer, MLitt. St. Paul, MN.

Printed by Bethany Press International, Bloomington, MN.

Cover by Elaina George, MD, and Dave Racer, MLitt

Second Edition

TABLE OF CONTENTS

"Every time I see a patient, I am reminded that I get to do what I love...and for that I am grateful to God."

– Elaina George, MD

DEDICATION

This book is dedicated in loving memory to my parents, Helen and Adolphus George, for their never ending love, support, guidance, and belief that I could do anything I set my mind to do. I love you both – thank you for everything.

ACKNOWLEDGEMENTS

Without the help and encouragement of many people, this book would not be possible.

I wanted to give a special thanks to Ms. Deidre Young for encouraging me to turn frustration and pain at watching a profession that I love be dismantled into an opportunity to speak out to empower both doctors and patients.

FOREWORD

As a third-generation physician, I am honored to be even a small part of *Big Medicine.*

My grandfather was a physician in Lima, Ohio. When he was debating whether to join the hospital staff in Springfield, over one thousand residents convened to beg him to stay. Of course he stayed. Not only did he continue his practice but established the Bradfield Community Center, a place to enrich the lives of low-income youth. The Center has quadrupled in size and is still operating eighty years later.

My father was a general practitioner in a low-income neighborhood. He charged his patients whatever they could afford. Then came Medicaid, the government program to finance medical care for certain individuals below the poverty line. My father did not accept Medicaid. Why? First, he could not afford to hire a second office worker to do the reams of paperwork and sit on the telephone following up Treatment Authorization Request forms. Second, charging patients on a sliding scale based on their ability to pay can be construed as health care fraud in the Medicaid program. The government managed to make charity a crime.

Slow forward to my own anesthesia practice that was the ultimate embodiment of price controls by the hospital and private and government insurers. In response to Hillary Clinton's attempted health care overhaul, I attended law school where I learned to decipher the administrative process. Working in health law, I witnessed how political wordplay shaped the increasing bureaucracy and dehumanization of medicine.

Over the last 40 years I have seen individuals receiving medical care go from being called "patients" to being health care consumers, clients, and treated like cattle. And in one of the biggest tricks played on the profession by health care hucksters, a physician is no longer your doctor. He or she has morphed into a nondescript generic fungible "provider."

Through my articles on our current issues in the delivery of medical care, I met a unique non-fungible woman – Dr. Elaina George. After listening to (and appearing on) her radio program, Medicine On Call, I became an instant fan.

Non-Fungible Doctor

Dr. George's patient advocacy begins with her medical practice that represents all the hallmarks of good old-fashioned medical care blended with the most advanced treatments – all at reasonable sliding scale pricing. She continues her activism by braving the netherworld of Washington, D.C. and appearing in the national media.

Big Medicine, The Cost of Corporate Control and How Doctors and Patients Working Together Can Rebuild a Better System is a labor of love. Dr. George has not merely cranked out yet another policy wonk book about our "health care system." Her journey through the health care maze provides an insight rarely seen. With every fact or figure, she reminds us that medical care is about human beings and should be approached accordingly.

Dr. George has performed an enormous service for patients and physicians. In straightforward and understandable language, Dr. George takes us on a journey through the gradual wrest of control of our medical care by politicians and large corporations who consciously disregarded input from independent private physicians – the backbone of medicine.

A Turning Point

We are at a turning point in the future of our medical care. Over time our concerns about "health care reform" have been confirmed: the Patient Protection and Affordable Care Act is about politics, not patients. Many were duped by buzzwords dripping with the lure of good health and at-the-ready medical care: "meaningful use," "accountable care organizations," and "medical homes." What we got was more gifts to corporate interests rather than substance offering a solution to high costs and accessibility. Clearly, centralizing control in the federal government and hiding costs through subsidies and middlemen – the insurers – is not the answer.

Dr. George channels her knowledge and medical experience into her prescription returning medical care to patient-centered delivery based on excellent care at a reasonable cost. Our responsibility as patients and physicians is to advocate for ourselves and insist that we maintain our medical privacy and individuality, the cornerstone of the patient-physician relationship.

Dr. George writes, "Liberty can only be preserved by people who pay attention and take action." A good first step is reading Big Medicine.

– Marilyn M. Singleton, MD, JD
June 2015

INTRODUCTION

By Dave Racer, MLitt

Big Medicine is the perfect title for a book
written by a solo practice doctor in the era of
the Affordable Care Act. Elaina George, MD,
is not unlike tens of thousands of physicians
who fight each day to preserve their liberty to
practice as they ought – not for themselves,
but for their patients. Dr. George's patients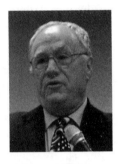
come first in her practice philosophy, but complying with the vo-
luminous and intrusive nature of federal regulations, piled upon
state and local regulations, added to the throes of operating a private business, has compounded her challenges.

Dr. George continues to focus on her patients, as she demonstrates
each day in her practice, because she knows it is the key to delivering quality health care. She uses every tool at her disposal, including offering medical services on a cash basis. She verbalizes
her arguments in the public marketplace of ideas in the hope that
somehow, some day, patient-centered healthcare provided by in-
dependently-thinking physicians, will once again become the
norm.

Dr. George asks a critical question: Why did President Obama, Congress, and the special-interest groups that helped them write the Affordable Care Act ignore the people who could have provided wise guidance as their new law came together? The solo practice doctor – and yes, doctors in a myriad set of practice models – have a firsthand understanding of how federal health policy affects individual patients. Instead, Obama and Congress turned to academia and activists – the results were predictable.

While no one can accurately predict the eventual ramifications of ObamaCare, as it has come to be known, one self-evident truth is that financing and delivery of healthcare is falling ever more to huge institutions.

> The five largest commercial health insurers in the U.S. have contracted merger fever, or maybe typhoid. UnitedHealth is chasing Cigna and even Aetna; Humana has put itself on the block; and Anthem is trying to pair off with Cigna, which is thinking about buying Humana. If the logic of ObamaCare prevails, this exercise will conclude with all five fusing into one monster conglomerate...
>
> Hospitals, doctors and other providers like rehab and skilled nursing are also uniting en masse. Irving Levin Associates reports that health services M&A deals rose 18% in 2014 after a record 2013...
>
> Hospital mergers have climbed every year since 2009, and in 2014 the number of deals that closed was 50% higher than the number in 2009, which was the year before the

health law passed. Three of five hospitals now belong to a
system. Hospitals are also absorbing physician groups, …[i]

The new complexity the ACA created in federalizing the disparate
U.S. healthcare system has overwhelmed the great and the small.
Health-provider systems of all sizes have been forced by the law
to spend thousands and millions of dollars in an attempt to comply
with ObamaCare's complicated and often contradictory demands.

Insurance carriers thought they would come out winners, or at least
worked day and night to make it so as Congress diced up their
products and dictated their new contracts. Caught in a whirlwind
of regulatory rollouts insurance companies have participated in a
futile attempt, while blindfolded, to throw darts at a moving target.
They have wasted billions on reforms that continue to be endlessly
reformed. There is no end in sight, until perhaps the final solution
becomes dissolution of the health insurance marketplace with one
or two massive Third Party Administrators simply managing the
federal governments' edicts.

The surest victims of a massively large, federalized, consolidated
healthcare system are individual patients and the tens of thousands
of independent practice physicians and surgeons who want to serve
them. More bluntly, patients have everything to lose in this gam-
ble that Big Medicine can deliver affordable, necessary, life-saving
healthcare for 320 million Americans (the third largest nation on
earth).

[i] Staff. (2015) ObamaCare's Oligopoly Wave. The Wall Street Journal. Washington, D.C.
6/19/2015 Retrieved 6/20/2015. http://www.wsj.com/articles/obamacares-oligopoly-
wave-1434755295

Big Medicine will be forever handicapped if it allows outliers to continue to practice medicine. It must eventually squash them. In many ways, the rollout of ObamaCare and previous federal legislation, has laid the groundwork for completely consolidating healthcare under the auspices of the all-knowing eyepieces of federal bureaucrats. This will have an unhealthy outcome for individual patients.

Elaina George says it did not have to be so. More so, she says it can be changed. It must be changed. Why? To save the medical profession? No. To do what healthcare systems are supposed to do – serve patients one at a time in a way that their medical condition requires.

This book will provide readers with the view that ObamaCare missed – that of doctors who look into their patients' eyes each day and work to reduce pain, suffering, and extend their lives. We patients depend on doctors doing the right thing for us, and that is why we need to free up physicians to be able to do so.

Thank you, Elaina George, for helping us better understand this.

Dave Racer, MLitt
Editor and Publisher

Chapter I:
Hippocratic Oath

It is hard to describe the feelings I experienced at the moment I finally could recite the Hippocratic Oath. It capped years of study and struggle to master complex science and even more complex people skills.

As with other contemporary movements that seem intent on destroying the profound nature of the human experience, even the Hippocratic Oath has a modern version that waters down key elements of the original Oath.

I recited the original version, translated to English. For physicians who are familiar with the Oath, you might want to move directly to Chapter 1. For others who are not familiar with the Oath, take some time to read the two versions. I suggest you read them aloud for the best effect. First, the "Classical" version, the one I recited and then the "Modern" version. You might be amazed at the difference, and by this understand some of the dilemma faced by the "healing arts" in our modern, nationalized healthcare system.

Classical Version:

I swear by Apollo Physician and Asclepius and Hygieia and Panaceia and all the gods and goddesses, making them my witnesses, that I will fulfill according to my ability and judgment this oath and this covenant:

To hold him who has taught me this art as equal to my parents and to live my life in partnership with him, and if he is in need of money to give him a share of mine, and to regard his offspring as equal to my brothers in male lineage and to teach them this art—if they desire to learn it—without fee and covenant; to give a share of precepts and oral instruction and all the other learning to my sons and to the sons of him who has instructed me and to pupils who have signed the covenant and have taken an oath according to the medical law, but no one else.

I will apply dietetic measures for the benefit of the sick according to my ability and judgment; I will keep them from harm and injustice.

I will neither give a deadly drug to anybody who asked for it, nor will I make a suggestion to this effect. Similarly I will not give to a woman an abortive remedy. In purity and holiness I will guard my life and my art.

I will not use the knife, not even on sufferers from

stone, but will withdraw in favor of such men as are engaged in this work.

Whatever houses I may visit, I will come for the benefit of the sick, remaining free of all intentional injustice, of all mischief and in particular of sexual relations with both female and male persons, be they free or slaves.

What I may see or hear in the course of the treatment or even outside of the treatment in regard to the life of men, which on no account one must spread abroad, I will keep to myself, holding such things shameful to be spoken about.

If I fulfill this oath and do not violate it, may it be granted to me to enjoy life and art, being honored with fame among all men for all time to come; if I transgress it and swear falsely, may the opposite of all this be my lot.[1]

Modern Version:

I swear to fulfill, to the best of my ability and judgment, this covenant:

I will respect the hard-won scientific gains of those

[1] Edelstein, L. (1943) Translation from the Greek by Ludwig Edekstein. From *The Hippocratic Oath: Test, Translation, and Interpretation.* Johns Hopkins Press. Baltimore, MD. 1943. Retrieved 1/29/2015.
http://hsl.mcmaster.libguides.com/content.php?pid=350076&sid=2920899

physicians in whose steps I walk, and gladly share such knowledge as is mine with those who are to follow.

I will apply, for the benefit of the sick, all measures [that] are required, avoiding those twin traps of overtreatment and therapeutic nihilism.

I will remember that there is art to medicine as well as science, and that warmth, sympathy, and understanding may outweigh the surgeon's knife or the chemist's drug.

I will not be ashamed to say "I know not," nor will I fail to call in my colleagues when the skills of another are needed for a patient's recovery.

I will respect the privacy of my patients, for their problems are not disclosed to me that the world may know. Most especially must I tread with care in matters of life and death. If it is given me to save a life, all thanks. But it may also be within my power to take a life; this awesome responsibility must be faced with great humbleness and awareness of my own frailty. Above all, I must not play at God.

I will remember that I do not treat a fever chart, a cancerous growth, but a sick human being, whose illness may affect the person's family and economic stability. My responsibility includes these related problems, if I am to care adequately for the sick.

I will prevent disease whenever I can, for prevention is preferable to cure.

I will remember that I remain a member of society, with special obligations to all my fellow human beings, those sound of mind and body as well as the infirm.

If I do not violate this oath, may I enjoy life and art, respected while I live and remembered with affection thereafter. May I always act so as to preserve the finest traditions of my calling and may I long experience the joy of healing those who seek my help.[2]

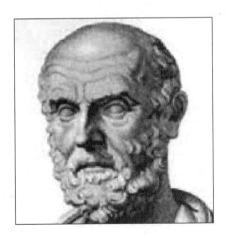

[2] Lasagna, L. (1964). Hippocratic Oath. Tufts University. Boston, MA. Retrieved 1/29/2015. http://hsl.mcmaster.libguides.com/content.php?pid=350076&sid=2920899

Ppaca & Hcera; Public Laws 111-148 & 111-152: Consolidated Print

One Hundred Eleventh Congress
of the
United States of America

AT THE SECOND SESSION

*Begun and held at the City of Washington on Tuesday,
the fifth day of January, two thousand and ten*

An Act

Entitled The Patient Protection and Affordable Care Act.

*Be it enacted by the Senate and House of Representatives of
the United States of America in Congress assembled,*

SECTION 1. SHORT TITLE; TABLE OF CONTENTS.

(a) SHORT TITLE.—This Act may be cited as the "Patient Protection and Affordable Care Act".

[Note: This print is of the Patient Protection and Affordable Care Act ("PPACA"; Public Law 111-148) consolidating the amendments made by title X of the Act and the Health Care and Education Reconciliation Act of 2010 ("HCERA"; Public Law 111-152). The text of the Indian Health Care Improvement Reauthorization and Extension Act of 2009 (S. 1790), as enacted (in amended form) by section 10221 of PPACA, is shown in a separate, accompanying document. This document has been prepared by the House Office of the Legislative Counsel (HOLC) for the use of its attorneys and its clients; it is not an official document of the House of Representatives or its committees and may not be cited as "the law". HOLC welcomes any corrections or suggestions to this document; these should be emailed to edward.grossman@mail.house.gov.]

(b) TABLE OF CONTENTS.—The table of contents of this Act is as follows:

Patient Protection and Affordable Care Act
(Later designated the Affordable Care Act)
Page 1 - Consolidated Version

CHAPTER 2
THE AFFORDABLE CARE ACT:
PATIENTS AND PHYSICIANS

Practicing physicians had no meaningful influence on the Affordable Care Act of 2010. From my perspective as a practicing physician, I see that patients likewise lacked input into ObamaCare – as it came to be known.

I felt that the time had come for a physician to explain the impact of the Affordable Care Act (ACA) on patients, and in a broader sense, on the United States' healthcare system. Hence, this book.

As a physician in private practice, I also see ObamaCare through the eyes of a small business owner. Physicians like me, who are self-employed or work in a self-owned clinic with partners, have all the obligations of business owners. We pay overhead expenses, manage employees, pay salaries, handle billings and collections, and have every tax obligation common to any small business. If governments change public policy that affects a business, it also affects a physician in private practice. What sets doctors apart from the hardware store, restaurant, gas station, or plumber is our professional responsibilities that directly affect life and death issues of our "customers" – patients.

My profession and my practice place me on the front line of health-care, directly serving patients. Over the past many years, my patients and I have experienced the devastating changes that have greatly affected the ability of an independent physician to deliver high quality healthcare. ObamaCare, however, is a special and far more dangerous encroachment than previous reform efforts. It has sped up, and continues to speed up the dissolution of the patient-physician relationship.

MD and Patient: Sacred relationship

ObamaCare, through its labyrinthine layers of regulations and regulators, intrudes on the sacred relationship between a patient and her/his physician. This one-on-one relationship is the most important aspect of efficient, cost effective, quality healthcare delivery.

I have been a practicing physician since 1998. Like most physicians since the earliest time of my life, practicing medicine is all I ever wanted to do. Initially, I wanted to be a veterinarian, but I couldn't stand the thought of seeing animals hurt or having to put them to sleep. Next, I wanted to be a cardiothoracic surgeon, and then, an orthopedic surgeon (since I played various sports throughout grade school and college). It is common among medical school students to take some time to settle on their lifetime passion. Finally, then, I selected ear, nose, and throat surgery as my specialty. ENT allowed me to be both a clinician and a surgeon. For me, ENT provided the perfect marriage of the essence of medicine – art and science.

Medical school professors taught us, as the first and foremost lesson, the primary importance of the physician-patient relationship. I learned that 90 percent of arriving at an accurate diagnosis started with collecting a thorough patient history, and getting a patient history meant talking directly with the patient. What a physician learns during the process of collecting this history goes far beyond mere collection of data. We pick up on verbal and physical cues, inflection, posture, and many more vital indicators than just the words spoken in answer to a question. This form of data collection requires the patient and physician to pay close attention to each other, and not to be distracted by the requirement of entering information on a computer while trying to listen – and see – what the patient is saying.

With the medical history in hand, I could then use the physical examination to confirm my diagnosis and use various tests to figure out the extent or progression of a disease. Getting the patient to reveal enough of the right information presented my greatest challenge, but it was essential in order to make an effective treatment plan.

Gathering medical history, examining the patient, assigning tests, and reading the results functions like detective work. Yet the physician must examine each case differently, with treatment options and plans tailored for the individual patient. Why? Because every human being is unique. While it is true that huge volumes of data about specific conditions can reveal common trends or diagnoses, the fact remains that each person responds individually to what medical science tells us to expect.

9

As a medical student, I remember writing up cases where two-thirds of my notes focused on the patient's history in his or her own words – I still do the same thing to this day. I can re-read my notes about a patient and remember everything I thought and felt at the time of each visit, because I made it my business to carefully listen to his or her story. I learned about the patient's family, the conditions that led them to make choices that have impacted them medically, and in some cases spiritually, so that I could treat the patient as an individual and not as a disease.

Enter the middlemen

Since I began my medical practice, I have seen changes incrementally forced on physicians that have fundamentally and dramatically affected our ability to provide high quality patient care. Today, providing care includes dealing with – and oftentimes fighting against – outside, non-medical forces. Insurance companies and multiple government agencies have become middlemen, standing like an impenetrable wall between physicians and patients. These third parties make decisions that hinder my ability to be an advocate for the best interest of my patients.

In many instances, these meddling middlemen have created an adversarial relationship between my patients and me. Their interference ruptures the trust relationship that is vital to successfully treating individuals. In place of that trust, the third parties attempt to force treatment options on us, and many are driven by actuarial decisions made by faceless entities that are only concerned with profit margins (private insurance) and/or cost savings (the Government). This leaves me to explain to a patient why a procedure can't be done, or why a medication will not be covered by insurance in spite of my professional judgment.

The actions of the outside middlemen have had a negative effect on the delivery of healthcare, driving up costs, limiting access to necessary care, and placing doctors and patients at odds with each other. Patients and physicians have long agreed that change had to happen. The United States' healthcare system had many flaws. We hoped that patients and physicians working together could control the outcome of change as it rolled out. Instead, Congress imposed a massive new oversized, top-down force on us in the form of a national bureaucracy of astonishing dimension.

When Congress passed ObamaCare in 2010 it severely exacerbated the problems with patient-physician medicine.

Reform of the wrong kind for the wrong reasons

In March 2010, Congress passed ObamaCare under the guise of caring for 50 million uninsured people. "Everyone will have health insurance," ObamaCare's proponents said. Those who had been shut out before would "gain access" to high quality, affordable healthcare. This was the message trumpeted across the country.

In reality, Congress designed ObamaCare to ensure that the worst aspects of the business of healthcare will proceed as usual. Under Congress' scheme, the corporate interests who advocated for ObamaCare will be well rewarded:

11

• Medical insurance companies gained a windfall of new subscribers who are mandated by government to pay higher premiums. ObamaCare does nothing to prevent insurance companies from continuing to put profits above patient care, increasing costs for patients through higher, and unaffordable out-of-pocket expenses (i.e., co-insurances, increasing deductibles and co-pays); limiting access to medical care through longer courses of medical management before a procedure can be done or a test can be ordered; expanding the practice of pre-certification of a medical test or procedure (e.g., getting prior approval); or outright denial of care despite the thousands of dollars the patient has paid in insurance premiums.

• Hospitals will become too big to fail. As the only game in town they will increasingly corner the market by becoming specialized centers of care or simply annexing community hospitals and private physicians under the guise of Accountable Care Organizations (ACOs). The increase in hospital-owned insurance plans will both limit the choice of where patients can receive their care and stifle local competition from private physicians, independent surgery centers, and smaller community hospitals which provide lower cost alternatives.

• The pharmaceutical companies win as they exercise heavy influence over evidence-based medicine. "Science" requires a pharmacological treatment, ordered by "evidence" from on high, rather than a procedure deemed proper by a physician and patient consulting together. Big Pharma stands to reap massive profits as ObamaCare touts "prevention," but really champions chronic disease management underwritten by medical treatment standards driven by research paid for by Big Pharma. Big Pharma will strive to reduce or remove competition from cheaper generic drugs and holistic therapies that rely on supplements and strategies that prevent or cure disease at a fraction of the cost of a brand name, prescription drug.

• The American Medical Association (AMA) represents perhaps as few as 15 percent of physicians nationally, but its influence extends into every medical transaction. It reaps hundreds of millions of dollars each year from its proprietary coding system (CPT coding) which all players in the healthcare system must use to communicate so that they can be reimbursed. AMA's political nature cannot be denied. In 2015 the AMA became the third largest spender in lobbying Congress, exceeded only by The US Chamber of Commerce and The National Association of Realtors. It is even more alarming when you know that although the AMA claims to represent the voice of physicians, the AMA only represents 1 in 5 doctors because physicians feel that the organization is out of touch with their needs and is in fact working against them. I am one of those who feels betrayed by the AMA.

Critical thinkers who care about the implications of public policy need to evaluate ObamaCare in light of this question: "Who stands to gain from the new law?" My experience shows that it is neither the patient nor the doctor.

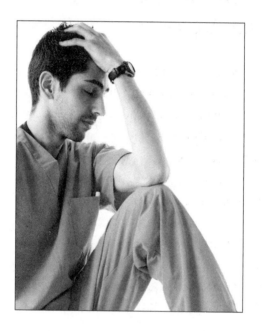

Chapter 3
Before ObamaCare,
Need for Reform

While there is much to dislike about the current system, wait until
ObamaCare is fully implemented. Our current healthcare system
suffers from the high price of medical care, expensive health insurance, and the needs for low-income people to be able to access
care; these need reform. ObamaCare does not resolve any of these
issues but, instead, will result in longer waiting times, increasingly
limited access for most people, ever more expensive insurance,
and reduced innovation. ObamaCare replaces doctor-patient medical care with an anonymous conveyor-belt style of medicine that
favors palliative over curative care. To the amazement of all, however, is the fact that you will be forced to pay more money for the
privilege of receiving less care.

At least since the 1930s, the United States has enjoyed the best
overall healthcare delivery in the world, but today, physicians on
the frontlines of medical care are watching it deteriorate. In my
opinion, the deterioration of our healthcare system is not an accident. Since Congress passed Medicare in 1965 we have witnessed
an incremental and well-designed plan to bring the U.S. healthcare
system down to the lower quality standards accepted by countries

with socialized healthcare. In short, ObamaCare, unless we can reform it, will complete our assimilation into a global, United Nation's driven socialized medical system.

ObamaCare is the fulcrum that will lock the U.S. in as the last piece of a socialized, single payer puzzle.

As I said earlier, taking the patient's history is the first step toward finding a treatment protocol. The U.S. healthcare system is the patient, and this book starts by explaining how we acquired our current condition. Then I will explain how we, as individuals, can learn the strategies and perfect the tools necessary to gain control of our personal healthcare choices. This is not a black or white issue; it is not a conservative or progressive issue; it is not a rich or poor issue; and it is not a male or female issue; this is not a racial or ethnic issue. ALL individuals want the same outcome – to be healthy, to live a long happy life, to love our friends and family, and to live in peace.

Each individual must exercise his or her God-given right to fulfill the talent that God has given to us. With that right, however, comes personal responsibility. When you have finished reading this book I am hoping you will have gained the will and knowledge to take back your power.

I am a physician, and it is all I have ever wanted to be. I love what I do. I recited the Hippocratic Oath when I became a physician, and it still means a great deal to me. As such, I want to empower patients and physicians to explore and celebrate the power that we have when we work together. The doctor-patient relationship is the foundation of excellent healthcare. If we start by honoring that relationship and move forward with courage and confidence, ObamaCare will wither on the vine.

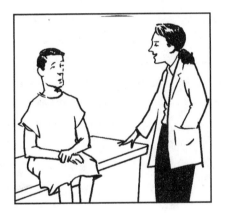

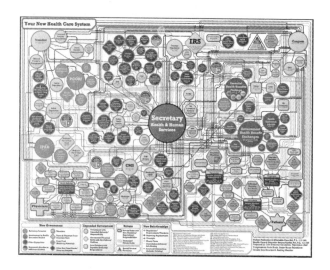

CHAPTER 4
ALONG CAME THE
AFFORDABLE CARE ACT
HR 3962 - THE HEALTHCARE REFORM
BILL: TRUTH AND CONSEQUENCES

A quick, but short history of the passage of what became known as ObamaCare is in order. First, voters gave Democrats control of the federal government in the 2008 election. Americans elected Democrat Barack Obama as President, and elected a Democratic Party majority of members in both the U.S. House and Senate. The House elected Nancy Pelosi, D-CA, as Speaker of the House. The Senate elected Harry Reid, D-NV, as Majority Leader.

President Obama tried to appoint former U.S. Senator Tom Daschle to be his Secretary of Health and Human Services. In 2008, Daschle had co-authored Critical: What We Can do About the Health-Care Crisis, with Nancy Lambrew. Daschle's book promoted the ultimate adoption of a government-run, single payer healthcare system. Unfortunately for Daschle, the media discovered he had failed to pay $128,000 in federal taxes and he had to step down. By his appointment, however, we can gain insight into what type of reform his boss, President Obama, preferred. Obama did appoint Nancy Lambrew to be a chief policy advisor on health-care reform, along with Ezekiel "Zeke" Emanuel, MD.

Zeke Emanuel had served at the National Institutes of Health for two decades. Zeke's brother Rahm Emanuel served as Obama's Chief of Staff. In 2010, Emanuel co-authored a much-heralded paper published in the Lancet, a world renowned medical journal. The article preached the virtues of the "Complete Lives System," for placing a financial value on human life as a means of determining who should receive care, when, and how much.

After Pres. Obama appointed former Kansas Governor Kathleen Sebelius as Secretary of Health and Human Services, the administration seemed set on trying to federalize one-fifth of the United States economy – the segment that provided medical care for 310 million people. With the Democratic Party firmly in control of the Congress and the Oval Office, the lawmaking began in earnest.

House passes radical bill

The healthcare reform bill (HR 3962) passed the federal House of Representatives on November 7, 2009 with a vote of 220-215. One Republican voted for it – Rep. Joe Cao of Louisiana. The bill was bad on so many levels it is difficult to fully explain.

As it stood at passage, it would have both destroyed the doctor-patient relationship and forever changed the practice of medicine as we know it.

HR 3962 eventually gave way to a Senate bill passed on Christmas Eve, 2009. Finally, on March 23, 2010, the Senate passed the so-called "Patient Protection and Affordable Care Act" (eventually labeled the "Affordable Care Act") and the House concurred. Several days later, Congress amended the Senate version of the bill so as to appease the left wing of the Democratic Party and their friends in the House.

There is great value and insight in reviewing the House's original intent to remake the U.S. healthcare system.

At the time the House passed HR 3962, we had one of the finest healthcare systems in the world. It had originally been built on the intimate relationship between a doctor and his or her patient, and a foundation of choice. Doctors were free to choose the care that they deemed necessary to treat their patients, and patients were free to seek the medical care of their choice. Although the capitation model of the 1970s and 1980s, with its attempt to limit medical spending by putting in place a primary physician gate-keeping system, had died a thankful death in the early 2000s, it had shaken the foundation and given rise to the powerful insurance-based third party payer system with its pre-certification, bundling of payments and cost shifting to patients in the form of higher out-of- pocket expenses.

During the decade of 2000-2010 modified versions such as the Health Maintenance Organization (HMO) and Point of Service (POS) plans which attempted to limit access to specialists thrived giving more power to insurance companies to make healthcare decisions. The insurers used the power of their anti-trust exemption to craft a system that produced monopolies whose primary purpose was to increase profits on the backs of both doctors and patients.

Unfortunately, when it passed HR 3962, the House failed to address necessary changes that would have led to meaningful reform. The starting point should have been to break the monopoly stranglehold that insurance companies still enjoy, and to reign in the enormous profits of the pharmaceutical industry. The House should have passed malpractice tort reform, or crafted a healthcare system based on wellness and prevention, and not disease management.

Instead, HR 3962 created a burdensome layer of new government bureaucracy that inserted itself between the doctor and the patient. It intended to create a national health commissioner and policy-making task forces to evaluate and decide everything from what medications a physician is allowed to prescribe to a patient, to what surgery will be approved, to what outcomes will be expected for a particular medical condition. It set up procedures to reward "good" physicians who followed government practice edicts with increased government reimbursements, and punish other physicians who had the audacity to challenge government-approved treatment protocols. It established the threat of severe fines for those who erred in completing its complex reporting requirements. In essence, it put physicians on the side of the line as a profession that needed watching and heavy-handed guidance.

Taken to its logical extent, HR 3962 would have created a world where the "good of the many," by definition, MUST outweigh the needs of the few. It presumed to limit spending large sums of money on a limited number of patients that might only serve to increase cost without the guarantee of a good outcome. Spending less on costly medical services only makes sense as long as you are not the senior citizen that needs a hip replacement, the premature infant with multiple medical problems, or the person with a chronic disease that statistics purport to show has a limited time left on this earth.

The House bill attempted to set up a healthcare system which presumed a finite number of resources (e.g., doctors, hospitals, expensive medical equipment). Given these presumed limitations, Congress decided that a government arbiter was needed to direct money to provide care to those whom the government determined to be the most productive people.

In 2010, Ezekiel Emanuel, MD, a senior White House health adviser, advocated for "The Complete Lives System" in the Lancet. This system prioritizes healthcare spending on younger to middle-aged persons on the theory that they have not yet lived a complete life and healthcare dollars would pay a higher return if invested in them, not in sickly children or unhealthy aging people. The system uses tools such as lottery and prognosis to determine who receives care.

The Complete Lives System leads us to a harsh reality. Those who passed HR 3962 saw it as an answer to the dilemma of how Amer-

ica can pay the medical expenses of more people with limited resources at a lower cost, and the bill's authors meant to do it without raising the federal deficit. The history of Medicare and Social
Security, both government-run programs, suggest that government
will be unable to keep its promises to provide care while, at the
same time, reducing costs to an expanding number of people.

HR 3962, however, served only as the dress rehearsal for passage
of the PPACA several weeks later.

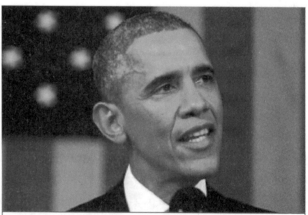

President Barack Obama's 2010 State of the Union
Address certainly caught my attention. I only wish
everyone listened carefully and took action.

CHAPTER 5
A PHYSICIAN'S RESPONSE TO THE
STATE OF THE UNION ADDRESS

*(I first wrote this as a blog entry after listening to President Barack
Obama's State of the Union Address on January 27, 2010. It has been
edited to make it timelier.)*

In his speech, which preceded the passage of the Affordable Care
Act by nearly two months, President Obama said:

> By the time I'm finished speaking tonight, more Amer-
> icans will have lost their health insurance. Millions
> will lose it this year. Our deficit will grow. Premiums
> will go up. Patients will be denied the care they need.
> Small business owners will continue to drop coverage
> altogether. I will not walk away from these Americans,
> and neither should the people in this chamber.

President Obama used his 2010 State of the Union Address to set
the stage for completing congressional action on healthcare reform.
In hindsight, and generally accepted today, it is easy to see how
the president and Congress mislead us about what they were doing
and its effect on the cost of insurance and access to care. As I
watched and listened to President Obama during that 2010 speech,

I considered the implications of what he promised, and now, what Congress eventually delivered.

The underlying philosophies of the Affordable Care Act included the idea that scientists and academics, cloistered under a government umbrella, could devise a reformed system of care and finance that would be a boon to everyone. The ACA, however, failed to take the most important thing into consideration – the relationship between the physician and his or her patient.

The right of an individual to choose his or her doctor (except in those rare instances when the patient is not sentient or mentally capable of making choices) should be inviolate. Furthermore, each individual, in partnership with a doctor, should be free to decide a course of treatment. The power of individuals to make informed choices about their own treatment is the foundation of excellent medical care. Under the provisions of the Affordable Care Act, however, the federal government has inserted itself into the doctor-patient relationship, becoming the final arbiter of individual medical care. This means that federal bureaucrats will ultimately decide who will become the health winners and losers.

Those who promote ObamaCare want people to believe that the U.S. healthcare system is so critically broken that it can only be fixed through comprehensive fundamental change with the government at the center. Because an ever increasing role of government is the answer to everything in this constituency, the rollout of ObamaCare was a win-win. The law's disastrous roll-out caused a chorus to argue for Medicare for all – a government-run single payer system. Both Senator Harry Reid and President Obama have been on record stating that that they favor a single payer system. In fact, however, an argument can be made that the government bailout written into the bill has actually already ushered in de facto single payer, as we see in practice that ObamaCare gives implicit or explicit control of healthcare expenditures to federal bureaucrats. Whoever controls the money controls access to care and makes the rules. With the ACA, the federal government controls the money and writes the rules.

Each day, since the ObamaCare train wreck rolled out (I paraphrase here Sen. Max Baucus, D-Montana, and the bill's chief Senate author), Americans are finding it painfully obvious that the ACA is not delivering quality healthcare. They're finding that having the right to insurance with no pre-existing conditions, "free" birth control, and preventive care paid at 100 percent, does not result in affordable care. They are looking at annual double-digit increases in insurance premiums for their mandated health insurance. They may not know it yet but although they may qualify for a premium tax subsidy, the IRS has the power to claw back some of those funds the following year if their financial situation improves – or they misstated their income on their application.

In those states that chose to expand Medicaid eligibility to 138 percent of income above the Federal Poverty Guideline, tens of thousands of individual are signing up for this "free" health plan.[3] Medicaid enrollees face a short-term and long-term challenge, and both could prove critical to their health and finances.

First, more than 50 percent of physicians refuse to take Medicaid patients because the reimbursements are too low. A doctor could go broke providing under-reimbursed care to too many Medicaid-covered individuals.

Second, later on when it's too late, an individual enrolled in Medicaid may find they will be unable to leave any of their wealth to loved ones. This is because state governments are allowed and encouraged to recover medical fees for payments made for their healthcare while on Medicaid – called "asset recovery." Over the prior years, states have collected tens of millions of dollars from the estates of deceased persons who had their healthcare provided at taxpayer expense. When Medicaid pays the bills, someday state governments will look to collect those tax dollar expenditures.

Another less discussed future problem with ObamaCare will be the cost to the taxpayer when the government stops picking up the bill to help states pay for Medicaid enrollees, leaving the states saddled with the bill. It is true that the ACA mandates the federal government to pick up 100 percent of the cost of Medicaid expansion at the outset, and 90 percent after 2017. No one, however, can guarantee that the federal government will have the money to continue to subsidize its share of Medicaid. When Congress is certain

---

[3] The federal government revises the Federal Poverty Guidelines (FPG) annually. The following are the income levels for 2015, at 138 percent above FPG. For individuals, $16,243; for a family of two, $21,238; for a family of three, $27,724; for a family of four, $33,465. These guidelines do not consider the dollar value of other welfare benefits that might be available to recipients (food stamps, rent subsidies, WIC, free meals, etc.), and to qualify for Medicaid under the ACA, the government ignores assets (property, savings, investments, etc.). Source: Medicaid.gov. Retrieved June 1, 2015.
http://www.medicaid.gov/medicaid-chip-program-information/by-topics/eligibility/downloads/2015-federal-poverty-level-charts.pdf

that Medicaid is fully-entrenched in the states, and realizes the federal government has no more money to make its 90 percent funding commitment, the states will inevitably stick it to the taxpayer to make up the difference.

As a result of the ACA, physicians are increasingly finding they will have little to no control over practicing the art of medicine. Doctors who practice under the auspices of the ACA will find themselves to be required to provide services deemed a patient's right that must be given for whatever value the government deems to be fair.

The ACA looks to huge organizations, such as Accountable Care Organizations (ACOs), to provide medical care on a capitated basis – a bundled payment of a set amount of dollars, determined by federal bureaucrats, for medical care that is split among the doctors, hospitals, clinics, pharmacies, and other medical vendors. The idea is in keeping with healthcare reformers' belief in the team approach to medicine. While there is great value in physicians collaborating with each other as their patient's medical needs demand it, the team approach is something different. The reformers mean to make doctors interchangeable with the healthcare team that includes non-physicians that provide care at a reduced price. Shifting the frontline of medical care to providers with 2-4 years of experience who were trained to be an adjunct to the physician will lead to the inevitable reduction in the quality of care, and it means we will see individualized healthcare and the art of medicine changed forever.

We must hope that before it is too late, Americans will come to the place where they know that the antidote to what is ailing the American healthcare system is NOT more government intervention, it is more choice via free market medicine. Yet, we can expect that each year, when this and future presidents give their State of the Union Address, we will hear more about how the federal government will solve the massive problems facing the delivery of and payment for healthcare for individuals. Unfortunately, we will hear little about improving the individual's right to choose their doctors and their course of treatment.

Chapter 6
Playing Politics Can Be
Hazardous To Your Health

Proponents of the Affordable Care Act claim one of their primary goals is to reduce healthcare costs. Immediately they began declaring victory because of the slowdown in the increase in total healthcare spending that we've seen in recent years. It's true that the annual increase in National Health Expenditures has slowed since 2007. What ACA advocates fail to mention is that far too many people are spending less because they can't afford to use medical services given the high out-of-pocket expenses common to ACA health insurance plans.

During each election season since the ACA passed we have seen that voters have remembered those members of Congress who voted for this disaster without having read the bill; those who demonized people who raised valid questions about access to care, costs and rationing. Voters remembered those Congressmen that cried racism when naysayers raised valid points about how the quality of and access to care would fall because the federal government does not have enough money to subsidize a substantial number of the 30 million newly insured people.

While voters may not know all the details about the ACA, their votes have shown they know it is the wrong solution, and they have continued to throw out of office those who cast Congressional votes for it – or forced early retirement on them.

Medicare enrollees need to remember that Congress took over $450 billion from the program – money that had been set to pay for the medical care of seniors – to fund the unwieldy ObamaCare bureaucracy.

ObamaCare promises to deliver cost savings, but instead, doubles down on what makes the U.S. healthcare prices so expensive – top down regulation. The ACA created a new bureaucratic infrastructure designed to transfer control of healthcare to central planners in Washington, D.C. The planners used innocuous catch phrases like "meaningful use," "accountable care organizations," and "medical homes." They point to "evidence-based medicine" as a panacea for affordable care. What these terms all have in common is they create a federal infrastructure to control the delivery of medical care. Central control achieves its goals by destroying the doctor-patient relationship and declaring which healthcare choices are allowed.

Now that we have had experience with the ACA's effects, it is becoming clearer that its promises have not been fulfilled, nor can they be. The primary promise, that you can keep your health insurance and doctor, has been shown to be a farce. Most often, people have not been able to keep their doctor or the health insurance they prefer. Instead, they have found themselves in slimmed down provider networks with few options, or enrolled in an Accountable Care Organization. The government has found ways to force those with a moral objection to abortion to pay for it, or spend tens of thousands on lawyers to defend their right to express their religious faith by refusing to fund abortion procedures.

The promised savings of $2,500 per family on health insurance premiums has morphed into thousands in premium increases, and potential family out-of-pocket expenses annually in excess of $13,200. Tens of thousands of employers have faced premium increases in excess of 40 percent, and some more than 100 percent. This has exposed their employees to an even greater cost of health insurance.

More than 220,000 doctors already refuse to accept ObamaCare's new Medicaid enrollees, a number that is growing. Doctors want to care for people, but because Medicaid reimbursements are so low they can't do so and keep their practices open. Furthermore, doctors, who believe in the Hippocratic Oath, have declined to accept new ObamaCare enrollees because they refuse to work against the best interest of their patients.

The decision to hide the true cost of health insurance – in premiums, out-of-pocket expenses, and loss of access – until after the 2012 election, was politics as usual. All that mattered to President Obama's campaign was winning his re-election, and trying to add more Democrats to Congress. Then as the 2014 election loomed closer, President Obama declared that the 2015 insurance premium increases would not be publicly disclosed until after the election.

To seal this deception, Obama declared that the open enrollment season would be delayed until November 15, instead of October 1, as the ACA law required. This type of politics reeks of cynicism and hypocrisy, and it shows the contempt that proponents of the bill have for the American people. It's been an ongoing pattern since Congress passed the ACA.

During 2014, the media began reporting how M.I.T. professor and economist, Jonathan Gruber, admitted that Congressional bill-writers viewed voters as stupid. Voters, apparently, are not as stupid as Gruber said. They threw out dozens of Democratic legislators and members of Congress during the 2014 election and elected the largest GOP House majority since the 1920s. Then they gave control of the U.S. Senate to Republicans. President Obama and his Democratic Party were, thereby, severely punished for their attempt to denigrate the world's best healthcare system.

- Even when individuals could keep their previous insurance, the premiums became more unaffordable. The increased out-of-pocket expenses have only added to this misery.

- More than 160 million Americans used to receive health insurance from their employers. As a result of the ACA, however, many smaller employers are dropping coverage because employers cannot afford it anymore.

The ACA's designers wanted to force individuals to enroll in medical insurance through government healthcare exchanges. By designing the ACA to pull the rug out from under individuals and employers, the planners expected it would leave individuals with no other options. Faced with an IRS-enforced mandate to purchase health insurance, and finding themselves without employer coverage, thousands flocked to federal and state health insurance exchanges, just as the ACA sponsors had hoped only to find themselves enrolled into government healthcare – Medicaid – or in subsidized health plans that still made medical care unaffordable.

Looking toward the future, as private insurance markets collapse, central planners hope to lead us into government-run, single payer healthcare. It is a plan that leads to the irreversible destruction of the essence of the United States' healthcare system, as it replaces individualized patient care with one-size-fits all, centrally-controlled care. If the ACA is allowed to take deep root, it will destroy the privacy and sanctity of the doctor-patient relationship. On each election day going forward, voters must continue to vote against ACA lawmakers, the only way to make sure it stops NOW. The voters sent a strong anti-ACA message through their Congressional choices in 2014. History will report whether the new Congress has had the courage to reform the ACA.

CHAPTER 7
IS ANYONE SEEING A PATTERN?

Americans tend to look at political and economic issues on an individual basis. We would do well to examine how each new Congressional initiative links to others, to see if a pattern exists. The Affordable Care Act may appear to stand alone, but it most certainly does not. It is part of a much larger pattern contributing to the power and influence of the federal government on individual lives.

Passing the ACA added yet another piece of the puzzle of a much larger picture to be put in place. A few months following passage of the ACA, Congress sent the Dodd-Frank "Wall Street Reform and Consumer Protection Act" to Pres. Obama. He signed it on July 21, 2010. Dodd-Frank, like the ACA, perpetuated a movement toward the national consolidation of power in a smaller number of large institutions, systematically removing free competition, and setting up the "too big to fail" phenomenon. These new laws, over the long run, will result in providing people with fewer banking and investment choices at an increased cost.

Consolidation of policy-making power at the federal level trickled down to consolidation at the local level – spurred on by the ACA. Since Congress passed the ACA, there has not been a lot of talk about the role that hospitals will play. The ACA, however, accelerated the shift of doctors from private practice to becoming hospital employees. All across the country specialty medical clinics have been bought out and merged with large hospital systems – the physicians most often become hospital employees. Many smaller community and doctor-owned hospitals have gone out of business as a result of ACA requirements, because they could not afford to keep their doors open under the new, onerous regulations.

There has also been a quiet consolidation of local hospitals. As hospitals have merged with clinics and other, smaller hospitals, they have become specialty centers for specific patient care. This also reduces patient choice.

It is not hard to visualize a future where there will only be a certain number of hospitals that are able to provide medical services for specialized diseases such as cardiac care, or orthopedic surgery. This specialization will limit competition in local communities so that access will be restricted – patients will be limited in choices of where to receive their care. For example, in a city or region with only one specialty heart center, that will create a shortage of cardiologists with a decrease in patient access. Simple math shows that with fewer doctors on staff, hospitals must limit the number of patients that can be treated at any specific time. Fewer specialists practicing at fewer facilities will likely lead to a de facto rationing of care.

Free market principles of competition based on supply and demand sets up a simple medical system that fosters excellence that is patient centered, since doctors will compete to offer patients the most advanced services at a reasonable cost in order to stay in business. An example of this is seen with plastic surgery and Lasik eye surgery. Both have traditionally been seen as cosmetic procedures, and therefore have not been covered by insurance policies. It may surprise many to know that the cost for procedures such as face lifts and tummy tucks have remained stable; and for popular procedures such as Lasik eye surgery, the costs have steadily decreased (when Lasik eye surgery was first introduced it cost as much as $10,000 per eye, now it runs from $250-$500 per eye).

The pressure of the free market has the power to control costs since costs are bound by what the market will bear. Price transparency trumps costs hidden in third party payer administrative bureaucratic fees which serve to exponentially and arbitrarily raise the cost of healthcare. Cost control is also strangled by hospitals which have increasingly become too big to remain efficient and now, too big to fail since removing small community hospitals and independent physicians.

Without competition among different hospital systems – or between formerly independent physician specialty groups – the price of medical services will likely increase. The large hospital systems have clearly pursued a strategy to organize themselves into non-competing systems which are the only game in town, removing any choice for the patient. When you add to the fact that they have begun to offer their own hospital-based insurance which locks patients into their hospital network because they won't cover out of network benefits, it is clear that they have become nothing more than medical cartels. With ObamaCare putting controls on what physicians are able to charge for the services that the government allows to be covered, the question of whether this cost containment strategy is good for the patient must be asked. I believe it is an emphatic "no!"

In 2008 we watched as Lehman Brothers collapsed, and then witnessed the merger of other large financial companies. This consolidation has led to very few winners in the financial industry – the biggest of which is Goldman Sachs.

The banking industry has seen a few surviving large institutions such as Chase and Bank of America. What the larger banks didn't acquire in mergers, the FDIC removed by taking over and closing hundreds of smaller and community banks. (It seems logical that the credit unions will be next on the list.)

Big Banking and Big Finance, with the help of the federal government, have not only survived but have also thrived, crushing their competition. Now it is Big Medicine's turn. The large hospital systems, now dominate the delivery of medical care in an increasing number of communities at the expense of the rural hospitals, which continue to close by the dozens.

Hospitals long have wielded power at state legislatures, and the ACA has strengthened their leverage. Hospitals are able to access government funds to pay for indigent care while private physicians are not. Despite this, in 2010 the Georgia Hospital Association tried to carve out an exemption for hospitals at the expense of physician-owned Ambulatory Surgery Centers (ASCs). Legislators had proposed a 1.45 percent "bed" tax on medical services to create a Medicaid fund. The hospitals tried to have language inserted into the bill to "protect hospitals from bills that are harmful to hospitals for three years" – effectively giving hospitals the power to "veto" any language in a bill that they didn't like. Doctors were not given access to the negotiating table, when the hospitals tried to get yet another Georgia law passed requiring that 2-4 percent of Georgia patients treated in private physician-owned surgery center must be indigent (i.e., physicians must treat indigent patients for free to keep their facility open), saddling private physicians with a competitive disadvantage since, in addition to this they still had to find the funds to pay all of the small business taxes, making it less likely that they would financially be able to remain open. Fortunately, enough physicians were able to contact members of the Georgia legislature to stop the hospital carve out. Had the hospitals prevailed they would have been in a position to further destroy competition from the private ASCs – and patients would have lost a less expensive alternative at which to receive care.

ObamaCare's authors made many bold promises; among them, was increased access to physicians. The more we observe the ACA's rollout the more we see how it limits patients' access to physicians, and how it results in fewer physicians in private practice. As the trend continues, the patient wait lines will increase.

This, then, is the Big Picture – the emerging pattern. Big Banking, Big Finance, and Big Medicine represent three of the pillars of an emerging nationalization of American life. The wise citizen would do well to be diligent about other efforts to nationalize American life – law enforcement and education, in particular. As this nationalization of life continues, each of us is left with greater taxes and fewer options – and with less liberty.

CHAPTER 8
THE APPOINTMENT OF DONALD BERWICK AS THE HEAD OF CMS

In April 2010, President Obama decided to appoint Donald Berwick, MD, to head up the Centers for Medicare and Medicaid Services (CMS). Seventeen months later, Berwick resigned, unwilling to face a potentially contentious confirmation hearing run by GOP Senate members.

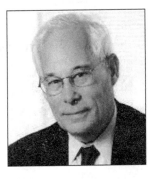

Berwick's appointment, however, provides insight into President Obama's intended goals of healthcare reform via the Affordable Care Act. ACA proponents had promised that healthcare reform would 1) mean better care for more people, 2) people would have more choice with more affordable healthcare and 3) individuals could keep the doctor and services that they wanted.

Berwick's appointment only clarified what many practicing independent physicians had already known – and which has been reinforced through various events since then. The ACA, like Berwick, intended to bend the cost curve at the expense of patients in the form of healthcare rationing. Berwick strongly supported pressuring doctors by limiting their individual ability to treat patients in the way they believed to be most medically sound.

During a 2008 talk Berwick delivered in the United Kingdom, he gave many insights into his belief system. Some of these bear repeating:

"I favor expanding choices. But, I cannot believe that the individual healthcare consumer can enforce through choice the proper configurations of a system as massive and complex as healthcare. That is for leaders to do."

Clearly, Berwick testifies to the Obama administration's nod toward centralized, top-down medicine in which the enlightened few would make decisions for the masses. This attitude is reflected in the tens of thousands of new regulations that have flowed from the CMS since passage of the ACA.

"I am romantic about the NHS [British National Health Service]. I love it."

In this, Berwick showed Obama's true colors and the long-term goals of the ACA. Obama himself had said, prior to running for President of the United States, that he favored a government-run, single payer healthcare system. It is a reason that many observers believe that the president hopes that as the ACA continues to fail, people will cry out for the federal government to take over the administration of healthcare for everyone; advocates often call this "Medicare for All."

"If a new drug or procedure is effective, and has some advantage over existing alternatives, then does the incremental benefit justify the likely additional cost?"

Clearly, Berwick felt no additional cost would be justified, even if it could be demonstrated as more effective.

His comments about the British National Institute for Comparative Effectiveness (NICE) should create chills in individuals living with chronic illness or suffering from serious medical complications; or for older individuals. "NICE is not just a national treasure; it is a global treasure," Berwick said.

The primary function of NICE is to decide the value of paying for an individual's medical treatment compared to the quality of life that is expected post-treatment. NICE looks at the value of spending money on medical care through a Quality Adjusted Life Years test. The NHS, under the NICE guidelines, would only spend healthcare dollars where NICE guidelines determine the financial reward justifies it. If the NICE guidelines determine that the QALYs from a medical procedure are too few for the money expended, then the medical care is withheld, although NHS might provide palliative care to make suffering and death more tolerable.

Despite their rigid attention to cost control, the rising costs of the United Kingdom's NHS has led them to become even more aggressive, instituting a recent guideline urging general practitioners to cold call seniors over age 74 and anyone, regardless of their age, with cancer, dementia, heart disease or a lung problem, to ask them to draw up end-of-life plans and do-not-resuscitate orders. One can only imagine the sound of ventilators beeping as plugs are pulled on patients all across America who end up on such a call list.

The United States Senate and Pres. Obama finally yielded to political pressure and Berwick left CMS before facing confirmation. He acknowledged that answering probing questions posed by Senators would not go well for him. More importantly, his answers would have revealed more than the Obama Administration would care to admit to at that point in time.

Berwick's attitude toward top-down managed healthcare, however, remains embossed in the ongoing rollout of the Affordable Care Act. The 2014 elections – finally – showed that this is clearly not the change that people were expecting or wanted. The question going forward is whether the new Congress has the will to fix the many flaws of the ACA.

CHAPTER 9
OBAMACARE IS A TROJAN HORSE FOR SOCIALIZED MEDICINE

ObamaCare is one of the most polarizing pieces of legislation ever passed by Congress. For proof of its polarization, look no further than the 2014 election results. Not only does the GOP House now have the greatest number of members in decades, but the GOP took over the U.S. Senate as well. All that holds the ACA in place is President Obama's veto pen.

Given its low ratings by voters, the question is how did its supporters pass this bill and where will it lead?

To pass the bill, ObamaCare supporters created a lot of political heat and blinded us with their rhetoric. They practiced identity politics, cultivated fear, ignited class warfare, stirred up racial animosity, and when all else failed, they simply lied. We heard that uninsured people were dying in the streets, a specious argument generated by a dubious study completed by David Himmelstein, PhD, and Steffie Wollhandler, MD, both of whom favor single-payer healthcare.

Another common charge made to radically overhaul the healthcare system was that greedy doctors were regularly performing unnecessary tests in order to run up their bills. Reformers declared anathema the idea of fee-for-service medicine, in which a physician charges a fee for a service performed, implying that doctors cannot be trusted. We heard a barrage of stories of surgeons amputating feet or taking out tonsils unnecessarily only to satisfy the doctor's unending quest to make as much money as possible.

As a counter argument to the manufactured "crisis" in access to and provision of U.S. healthcare, we heard that without ObamaCare, our healthcare system would collapse.

When ObamaCare supporters claimed uninsured people could not get healthcare, they lied. There are many proofs of their lie. Among them is the fact that because of the Emergency Medical Treatment And Active Labor Act (EMTALA) passed in 1986, a hospital emergency room cannot deny care to anyone in this country, whether a citizen or not. Congress meant for EMTALA to provide an open door to an uninsured person in need of emergency services. Unfortunately, this unfunded congressional mandate led to the unintended consequence of people using the emergency medical system for primary care. Hospitals, even non-profits, despite having access to government money set aside to pay them to cover these patients, have continued to pass along the cost of delivering "free" healthcare to paying customers – essentially double dipping. This contributes to the explosion in the cost of hospital care. EMTALA is a perfect example of how government intervention has been the chief contributor to soaring hospital costs. Instead of fixing this,

ObamaCare left EMTALA in place and as we see it now. Another failure of ObamaCare is the fact that even more people are using the emergency room for care because they can't afford the high out-of-pocket costs of premiums, deductibles and co-insurance that have steadily risen since its implementation.[4]

ObamaCare's supporters seldom if ever talked about the thousands of public health clinics, many funded through private donations. We saw no media mention of free healthcare clinics in which thousands of physicians provided services at no cost to uninsured persons. Neither did ObamaCare supporters acknowledge the thousands of hours of voluntary uncompensated care provided by physicians and surgeons. Also lacking in media coverage were the stories of emerging private market initiatives to provide healthcare services at a low or reduced cost.

ObamaCare supporters and their media allies repeated the uninsured meme to such an extent that it became a "truth." Moreover, they translated the idea that lacking a health insurance policy or lacking enrollment in Medicaid or some other government program meant that uninsured people could not access healthcare. (Going without enrollment in some form of a health plan is not a good idea. It would be good if 100 percent of American residents could insure themselves against large medical losses, but that is different from ObamaCare's goals.) The problem is that Oba-

---

[4] Cunningham, P. Does ObamaCare make insurance cost too much? The Washington Times. Washington, D.C. May 15, 20105. Retrieved June 1, 2015. http://www.washingtonexaminer.com/does-ocare-make-insurance-too-costly/article/2564541

maCare supporters did not tell the whole truth, and their plan to fix the partial truth has come up completely short.

Serving to divide and conquer opponents, mainstream media demonized anyone who questioned the motives or facts of the ObamaCare reformers. Often – far too often – supporters and media allies attempted to muzzle ObamaCare detractors by playing the race, class, and/or immigration cards. Those who opposed a federal takeover of healthcare were accused of discrimination against all manner of minorities. Media dismissed ObamaCare critics as part of the problem, as those who favored Big Pharma, Big Medicine, and Wall Street over the best interest of the people.

Meanwhile, as usual, a deafening silence emanated from medical professionals who serve on the front lines. The professional associations that represent physicians and surgeons, almost in unison, fought to get a "place at the table," as Congress rolled through its ACA bill-writing exercise. Getting a place at the table, so thought these short-sighted leaders, meant making sure that once the federal government completed its coup over medicine, at least the organization's members could keep on working in healthcare or health finance. Instead of putting patients first, too often the special interest groups put their own association's survival first. It is easy to see why we are where we are now. And where are we? We sit on the brink of dropping into a global healthcare delivery system driven by rationing based on:

1)   Long waiting times leading to limited access to care.

2)   Limited access to medical innovation.

3)   An emphasis on the management of chronic disease.

4)   End-of-life decisions based on limited intervention with an emphasis on palliative care not curative care.

Filmmaker Michael Moore released his movie, "SiCKO" in 2007. He purported to show how far better healthcare was in foreign nations. "A documentary comparing the highly profitable American healthcare industry to other nations..."[5] Moore withheld the truth. He could have told the audience that The National Health Service (NHS) in Britain is going bankrupt. NHS managers have, in fact, considered hiring a German company to manage it, and recently had a hospital system taken over by a private management company. Furthermore, that the NHS has changed the guidelines for treatment of diseases such as glaucoma and ventilation tubes for ear infections, and procedures like knee replacements, making it more difficult for patients to qualify for the procedures.

The NHS considers the gold standard of cancer care to be met when a woman is able to see an oncologist within two months of diagnosis for breast cancer. The UK suffers from a severe lack of oncologists, so not only are wait times longer than in the U.S., but mortality is also higher.

When the U.K. launched the National Health Service in 1948, its founder stated that the system could never provide the volume of healthcare people would want to use. It proudly declared there

[5] IMBD. "SiCKO" Retrieved 2/12/2015. http://www.imdb.com/title/tt0386032/

would be no co-pays, deductibles, or out-of-pocket cost, but by 1952, began charging small co-pays. By 1989, the UK authorized the issuance of private health insurance to meet the care gap created by shortages at all levels of care. More than 13 percent of UK residents opted out of the government-run, NHS by 2005.

Why would anyone want the United States to move toward the limited care options available under a government-run healthcare system? But that is precisely the direction taken under the Affordable Care Act.

Powerful Opted Out Early

It is galling that members of Congress, corporations like McDonald's and Cigna Healthcare, and the unions who were all proponents of the bill will not have to live under its yoke, at least at its outset. Instead, they won reprieve at the behest of the Department of Health and Human Services under Secretary Kathleen Sebelius. Instead of a predictable public policy setting equal rules for everyone, we saw raw politics as the DHHS applied rules unequally, favoring their friends. This lends testimony to the idea that the folks who "know what is best for us" also think they know who is required to follow the rules, and what the rules should be.

For a variety of reasons which we will continue to unwrap in this book, ObamaCare does not deliver efficient, affordable healthcare, but instead it sets up a complex system of top-down control based on the creation of manufactured scarcity:

1. Not enough doctors to deliver care.

2. Not enough hospitals to care for the 30 million more people who allegedly will access the system.

3. Mandates which lock individuals into a system that strips away their choice while making them pay for the privilege.

4. Bureaucratic panels which micro-manage the entire healthcare system while establishing a plethora of regulations that demand compliance in the face of penalties for those who dare to buck the system, or who make mistakes.

5. Prohibitive costs, finally admitted to, that are the outgrowth of the oversight needed to police this Draconian system.

Unworkable Paradigm

The ObamaCare system is financially unsustainable. Its poor planning is built on a foundation of "one-size-fits-all" that will bankrupt our country or destroy the quality of American healthcare – or both. ObamaCare will grow ever-larger and more corrupt while perpetuating and rewarding the worst aspects of corporate healthcare. President Obama's term expires at Noon on January 20, 2017. Tens of thousands of pages of regulations will be enforced by then, and ridding ourselves of their shadow will be difficult, if not impossible.

This is an example of the problem, reaction, and solution paradigm:

1. Problem: Once people realize what they will really be getting, they will know it was not what they signed up for and there will be massive outrage.

2. Reaction: They will demand the government to step in and fix it.

3. Solution: Government-run, single-payer healthcare.

And there you have it. After years of sidestepping the truth, Americans may be perfectly set to accept socialized medicine; but maybe that was the goal all along.

CHAPTER 10
CRONY CAPITALISM CAN BE
HAZARDOUS TO YOUR HEALTH

Michael Moore, the moviemaker, pontificated in the past that under ObamaCare, Americans would have to wait to receive care for certain non-life-threatening procedures such as a knee replacement. Moore believes a "patriotic American" would be happy to wait. If Moore took the time and made the effort to take a critical look at socialized healthcare, he would see the obvious fact that it doesn't work, and in fact, it hurts people.

Moore and his ilk talk of healthcare equality. By this they mean that everyone should be able to get every medical procedure they need at someone else's expense. Real life experience around the globe suggests that Moore is deluded. Despite Moore's pronouncements, because of ObamaCare, America is rapidly moving toward a two-tier medical delivery system that is separate and unequal – one system, provided for by government and paid mostly by taxpayers and another, private system paid for by those who have the means to do so. Those who can afford to pay their own way, as they do in the United Kingdom, will simply opt-out of government care.

Through the Affordable Care Act, politicians have imposed government onto our healthcare system and created the position in which we increasingly find ourselves. Cronyism has given corporate interests such as Big Pharma, medical insurance companies, and hospitals, the power to systematically remove competition, control prices, and lead to a too big-to-fail phenomenon. These deliberate political decisions have left doctors and patients on the outside looking in, dependent on "those who know what is best for us" to decide what it means to provide appropriate care. We watch aghast to see these forces continue to gut what was once the best medical system in the world.

The medical insurance industry lobbied heavily to pass ObamaCare. Why? America's health insurance companies expected to gain more than $40 billion in new annual premiums, much of it underwritten by taxpayers. The insurance companies see themselves as an example of an ObamaCare supporter that will be a big winner.

Michael Moore can make easy pronouncements about patriotism and duty to wait for care all he wants (he also has a fortune to help pay for his own care), but the reality is that already, just a few years after passage of the ACA, people are already suffering because of delays or being denied medical procedures. Physicians are put in the untenable position of watching their patients suffer needlessly, and in some cases, die because insurance companies deny care they deem to be medically unnecessary, or the patient simply cannot afford the out–of-pocket costs of their deductibles and co-insurance. How does this happen?

Physicians who receive reimbursements for care from Medicare, Medicaid, or insurance companies are at the mercy of these payers. The payers require physicians to gain pre-approval for a good deal of care, or the insurance company gate keepers decide against re-imbursing other forms of care. They use "science-based" guide-lines to instruct physicians what to do under various circumstances. Taken together, the physician's ability to direct the medical care of a patient is stripped away, and given to others.

As physicians, we take an oath to do no harm. Sometimes it seems that after taking the Hippocratic Oath we take another oath – to keep quiet.

Physicians have to understand that healthcare is now subject to elective politics and advocacy by interest groups. This means that for the sake of our patients, we have to speak out. We are respected in our communities; people will listen to us if we can communicate our advocacy for patients. One of the greatest harms we do is to re-main quiet. Physicians need to explain what is happening to their patients, and together, they must make their voices heard before individual choices are legislated away.

We are beginning to see that ObamaCare will potentially put more people in an increasingly broken system that will systematically delay and deny care all in the name of cost savings for the false feel-good meme of universal coverage.

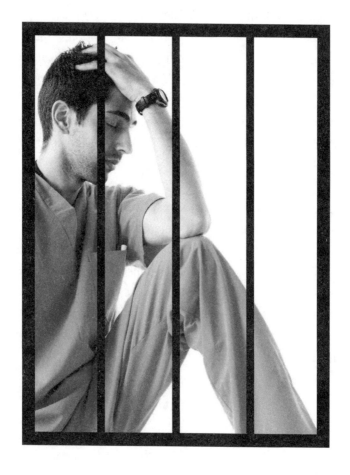

Chapter 11
ObamaCare Endgame:
If Doctors Choose to Put Patient Care First, they Can Look Forward to Fines or Jail Time

If federal officials and their cronies in the 50 states completely implement ObamaCare, doctors will no longer be practicing medicine. Instead, doctors will become like drones, managed by the "joy sticks" of distant government and third party bureaucrats who determine their course of treatment. In the ObamaCare nirvana, doctors are tasked with doling out the meager healthcare crumbs authorized by the bureaucrats who hold the ultimate power over an individual patient's life – or death. This will become all too clear when it is, perhaps, too late to change as individuals with medical conditions that require treatments which the bureaucrats have determined not to be cost effective, will receive a one way ticket to a hospice.

Early on, even before Congress passed ObamaCare, we could see the Obama Administration ramping up its efforts to control the distribution of medical services. Congress used a common strategy when dealing with what should be a controversial issue; Congress hid provisions in the 2009 "stimulus bill" that reduced citizen scrutiny about to what Congress' really intended to do. The 2009 "Stimulus" bill appropriated $1.1 billion to create an important piece of the framework for the healthcare bill, money that funded the Coordinating Council on Comparative Effectiveness Research. The Council intended to use studies largely underwritten and sponsored by Big Pharma that they consider "science" to endorse treatment protocols it believes to be appropriate, and to dismiss those it does not endorse. Besides being used to determine when or if a doctor is paid to provide a service, the end result is truly to decide whether an individual patient will receive medical treatment. The false concept on which the Council bases its edicts is that doctors, in consultation with their patients, don't have the ability to make correct healthcare choices.

Comparative effectiveness is taken somewhat from the United Kingdom's National Institute for Comparative Effectiveness – misnamed "NICE." We discussed NICE earlier. In summary, NICE helps determine the value of a human life when compared to expected medical outcomes. Based on this formula, the NHS determines how much, if any, additional care a person will receive.

After Congress passed ObamaCare, we began to learn about the Independent Payment Advisory Board. The IPAB consists of 15 people appointed by the President. They share a common characteristic – they are isolated from day-to-day patient care. How can such a Board make any valid decisions about the real practice of the art of medicine? The Board, like NICE, is tasked with something far different – it is to evaluate patients as a cost center that

needs to be controlled. With advocates of the "Complete Lives System" guiding its decisions – consultants like Dr. Zeke Emanuel –
it is hard to ignore the probability that senior citizens, individuals
with chronic illness, and the very young who appear to or have real
physical abnormalities, will be sent to the outside of America's
healthcare system and left to look in, bereft of necessary medical
care. The IPAB is another example of the people of this country
being told by the government that it knows what is best for us.

The stimulus bill funded the framework to set the stage for the implementation steps found in ObamaCare. The law used fear and
intimidation to force doctors to comply. Continuing what the Stimulus Bill started, ObamaCare intimidates doctors to, a) willingly
destroy the doctor-patient relationship, b) and to betray their Hippocratic Oath to provide treatments that they deem to be effective.
Steven Brill in his book America's Bitter Pill, showed how ObamaCare's creators had disdain for the "sacred physician-patient relationship" and considered it to be mere marketing tactics by the
anti-ObamaCare forces.[6] Any doctor can easily dissuade you of
such nonsense: If patients cannot trust doctors to do what doctors
believe is best, the patient's health will suffer, as will the entirety
of the traditional way we deliver healthcare in the United States.

The stimulus bill created a second board, called The National Co-
ordinator for Health Information Technology. Its purpose is to "…
determine treatment at the time and place of care." The board
members are charged with deciding the proper course of treatment

[6] Brill, S. (2015) America's Bitter Pill. Random House, New York.

for a doctor's diagnosis. Given the plainly-stated purpose of this federal information technology, it is obvious why government-managers have made a big push toward the mandatory implementation of universal electronic medical records (EMR).

These EMRs potentially give federal regulators direct access to each patient's private medical records and at the very least, tie together the records of any single doctor into a unique individual provider data base. Armed with this information about each doctor – and patient – central planners will have the hook they need to completely control the physician and the patient. Government-managers, in the statutes, rules, and regulations show how they will be able to punish physicians and hospitals. Those physicians that choose to practice individualized care in consultation with their patients and refuse to succumb to interoperable EMRs will be fined for not being "meaningful users of the system over time." In the original ACA as passed, since January 1, 2013, every doctor has felt the weighty threat of a $100,000 penalty for not installing and signing on to government-mandatory EMRs and instead, doing what he or she believes is the right thing for a patient – and this is for a first "offense." Doing what is right a second time, in defiance of the central medical planners, could land a physician in jail.

The threat of fines, penalties, and prison has many perverse effects on physicians and patients. Forced to conform to federal edicts, the physician will no longer be able to practice medicine as he or she believes in the best interest of patients. The mere threat of retaliation by bureaucratically-prescribed medical practices will have a chilling effect on physicians. It may be the straw that completely breaks the foundation of good medicine – the doctor patient relationship.

Prior to ObamaCare's passage, 46 percent of surveyed physicians told The New England Journal of Medicine that they would leave the practice of medicine if ObamaCare was implemented. Merritt-Hawkins' 2014 survey of physicians, conducted five years later, saw that number of physicians who expected to retire fall to 38.6 percent. Perhaps thousands had already done so between surveys, but 38.6 percent still represents hundreds of thousands of doctors.[7] Furthermore, 45.8 percent of doctors felt the EMR detracted from providing efficient medical care, and only 4.6 percent saw EMRs as improving interaction with patients.[8]

When ObamaCare passed in 2010, planners expected 30 million more patients to enter the healthcare system. Lawmakers knew this doctor shortage posed a real threat. Instead of reducing disincentives for doctors to practice, such as federally-monitored interoperable EMRs, Congress made a big push to increase the number of other types of providers, such as physician assistants and nurse practitioners.

With ObamaCare in place, there is no question among doctors that healthcare rationing will become our future. Adding 30 million

[7] Merritt Hawkins Staff. (2104) 2014: A Survey of America's Physicians: practice Patterns and Perspectives. The Physicians Foundation. Boston, MA. September 16, 2014. Retrieved 3/28/2015. http://www.physiciansfoundation.org/news/survey-of-20000-u.s.-physicians-shows-80-of-doctors-are-over-extended-or-at

[8] Ibid.

more people enrolled in government-paid Medicaid into a system now shackled by reduced resources makes it impossible to avoid rationing. Perhaps those members of Congress who passed this nightmare didn't care since they made sure that it wouldn't apply to them.

CHAPTER 12
IN THE AGE OF OBAMACARE,
WILL YOUR MEDICAL INFORMATION
BE USED AGAINST YOU?

Since 2010, when Congress passed ObamaCare, the public has been preoccupied with the fear of a government takeover of health-care, but maybe this is the wrong focus. Perhaps we should be just as concerned about a corporate takeover of healthcare.

President Bill Clinton signed the Health Information Portable Ac-countability Act (HIPAA) into law in 1996, ostensibly to protect each individual's medical privacy. "The HIPAA Security Rule es-tablishes national standards for the security of electronic protected health information." The federal government required all covered entities – health plans, doctors, hospital and other healthcare providers, as well as third party administrators – to comply by April 14, 2003.[9] HIPAA's proscriptions were ostensibly intended to pro-tect patient privacy through a complex system of regulations en-forced by the federal government. These regulations amount to promises not kept, exemplified most recently by the cyber-attack

[9] Staff. (2015). Enforcement Highlights. Centers for Medicare and Medicaid Services. Washington, DC. http://www.hhs.gov/ocr/privacy/hipaa/enforcement/highlights/

which caused a breach of private health information from Blue Cross - Blue Shield.

HIPAA interpretation and application has created a legal club for regulatory enforcers and laid on yet another layer of federal control over the delivery of and payment for healthcare. Federal HIPAA bureaucrats impose costly fines on physicians, and violations can result in jail time. HIPAA gave bureaucrats powerful tools to punish those who government has deemed are violating its rules. HIPAA created an entire new industry of healthcare compliance consultants, attorneys, and administrators. This is another example of the asymmetric use of coercive power against the physician. After its data breach, Blue Cross only had to apologize and promise to do better next time, a luxury not afforded a physician. The physician that accidentally releases patients' records into the "Cloud" can expect fines leaving him or her bankrupt, and time spent in jail.

The Recovery and Reinvestment Act of 2009 gave the Secretary of the Department of Health and Human Services the power to determine the amount of fines and whether civil penalties will be applied to those who violate HIPAA. This enforcement exists outside of ObamaCare and is another example of a legislative sleight of hand. As lawmakers created ObamaCare they knew that, combining the HIPAA law and regulations already in place, with its threats of fines and penalties, they had no need to include its enforcement procedures in ObamaCare. This is a cruel but typical strategy Congress uses to slide in questionable, unpopular processes without the public's knowledge.

Within weeks of passing ObamaCare, big corporations and unions realized they had set a trap for themselves by supporting the new law. As a result, then Health and Human Services Secretary Sebelius granted waivers to thousands of big corporations such as Google.com, Waffle House, and Foot Locker, and supporters of ObamaCare such as Aetna, Cigna and the SEIU. The Secretary's actions sent a signal to doctors that those who oppose the administration needed to watch their backs and would not receive special treatment or relief.

The Washington Times published an article by Milton Wolf, MD, titled "The Tawdry Details of ObamaCare," that provided an excellent synopsis of the privileged treatment bestowed upon friends of the administration. Wolf wrote, "It was Mr. Obama himself who infamously said, 'We're gonna punish our enemies and we're gonna reward our friends.' This president speaks anything but softly, and ObamaCare is his big stick."[10] Those who were not lucky enough to receive these insider waivers faced the thankless task of being under the mandate's yoke and, therefore, picking up the tab. In an age where politicians constantly talk about "fairness," how fair is that? This is yet another example of rules that are unequally applied.

When Secretary Sebelius granted a waiver to Google it led one to wonder what other favors would the administration grant to Google, if not now, at some time in the future? Big Data will be pressing toward a way to use the massive database generated by

[10] Wolf, M, MD. (2011) Tawdry details of ObamaCare. The Washington Times. Washington, DC. 1/28/2011.

ObamaCare reporting requirements, and Google seems like an obvious choice to exploit this potential.

It is conceivable that Google (or another mega-data processing company) will be able to find and use a loophole in HIPAA to flout the regulations and share or sell any individual medical information that they might obtain through any number of sources. On June 24, 2011, Google announced that they were discontinuing their Google Health Website that they launched during May 2010. Google had stated in their privacy policy that they would not sell private health information, but Consumer Watchdog charged that, on the contrary, Google had lobbied Congress to allow them to do just that. If Congress had allowed this exception, Google would have joined pharmacies and pharmaceutical companies in the ability to make a profit off private health information. Citizens must keep a close eye on the purveyors of Big Data, like Google as it seems inevitable that someday, they will be marketing private health information as they now market books, cab rides, and vacations.

In explaining their decision to drop the service, Google wrote:

> In the end, while we weren't able to create the impact we wanted with Google Health, we hope it has raised the visibility of the role of the empowered consumer in their own care. We continue to be strong believers in the role information plays in healthcare and in improving the way people manage their health, and we're always working to improve our search quality

for the millions of users who come to Google every day to get answers to their health and wellness queries.[11]

Furthermore, granting any corporation the freedom to sell your private information opens up the possibility that government bureaucrats and planners would have direct access to your specific health information. A Big Data company could conceivably share your information with employers, political adversaries, or government agencies such as Medicare or the National Security Agency. For example, if you put on your form that you had some medical condition or habit that you declined to disclose to your doctor, you may unknowingly be sharing that information with insurance companies, the many number of government agencies or anyone with the reason or wherewithal to purchase it.

In short, the United States government could hold Google or any Big Data company to a different standard from that which it holds a physician. Since Big Data companies are not limited by the strict confidentiality requirements of the doctor-patient relationship, they might be read to share health data for the right price.

If a doctor discloses private medical information to government agencies, he or she could be fined up to $250,000 and potentially be imprisoned up to 10 years. The Department of Justice broadened the definition of potential violations, so that a federal prose-

[11] Staff. (2011) an update on Google Health and Google PowerMeter. June 24, 2011. Retrieved on March 30, 2015. http://googleblog.blogspot.com/2011/06/update-on-google-health-and-google.html

cutor can now charge a physician for violating HIPAA even though the doctor has no knowledge of the specific violation. In this way, federal prosecutors would now view the physician as guilty until proven innocent. This is a recent DOJ interpretation of the criminal breach of HIPAA regulations: In defining "Knowingly," the DOJ interpreted the "knowingly" element of the HIPAA statute for criminal liability as requiring only knowledge of the actions that constitute an offense. Specific knowledge of an action actually being in violation of the HIPAA statute is not required when deciding whether to prosecute an individual.

Google offers an example of the growing list of companies that have a creepy connection to the federal government. Like the Food Safety Modernization Act, SB 510/HR 2751, which became law in January 2011, which attempted to give control of our food supply to Big Agra, in the same way, the Healthcare Reform Bill has given control of our healthcare system to Big Pharma, insurance companies, and corporate hospitals.

This cozy relationship between Google and federal bureaucrats appears to be yet another attempt to insert a corporate middleman between us and our right to privacy. First it's the carrot, then the stick: The idea of storing your medical history at Google or any other Big Data company is attractive, and you would do it voluntarily. Then, like other social media websites, you will find yourself in a position where it can be used against you.

ObamaCare has put all of us in additional jeopardy from the potential that our private medical data will be shared with government agents and others with whom we disapprove. This is wrong and can serve no purpose other than to denigrate our precious individual rights and liberty.

CHAPTER 13
THE ANTIDOTE TO THE AFFORDABLE CARE ACT, AND A MISGUIDED SUPREME COURT, IS NON-PARTICIPATION

On June 28, 2012, the United States Supreme Court (SCOTUS) issued its decision on NFIB v. Sebelius. SCOTUS releases scores of decisions each year and most often, there are a relatively small number of people or institutions that pay attention. NFIB, however, held the attention of hundreds of thousands of Americans and scores of big-money interests, not to mention everyday Americans. If the Court decided that ObamaCare's individual mandate was unconstitutional, it would bring the health insurance industry to its knees. Doctors, hospitals, clinics, third party payers, Pharma, medical device companies, and other medical providers would have been forced into a mad scramble to protect themselves from an onslaught of uninsured individuals needing medical attention.

Most conservative court-watchers, and not a few liberals, felt certain a 5-4 decision would result in repeal of the individual mandate as an abuse of the Commerce Clause by Congress. SCOTUS did issue a 5-4 decision, but it upheld ObamaCare, and the swing vote to keep it in place came from a presumably conservative justice, John Roberts. Roberts' troubled logic reframed the debate from an overreach of the Commerce Clause to the right for Congress to levy taxes. Roberts saved ObamaCare by calling the mandate to purchase insurance a tax, and ruled it to be an enumerated power granted to Congress by the Constitution.

The SCOTUS' NFIB decision, paradoxically added pressure to the inevitable slide to end patient-driven healthcare. Healthcare that is patient-driven can only occur through individualized medicine led by independent doctors in consultation with a patient. The ACA, on the other hand, views healthcare as system-driven, with central planners making decisions on behalf of individual patients who are members of "populations," using doctors to deliver their "science-based" edicts.

The SCOTUS' NFIB decision, however, did not represent a breakthrough in thinking about how we do healthcare financing. The foundation for our modern insurance system had been laid decades earlier. We need to understand how we came to this juncture, in how we finance the practice of medicine and how it affects the delivery of care, to learn what needs to be done to get out of this situation.

How did this get started?

In 1971, the U.S. Department of Health, Education, and Welfare (HEW) funded the Rand Health Insurance Experiment – a study conducted by the Rand Corporation. The report that came from this study planted the seeds from which rose today's health insurance companies. The Rand study concluded that by increasing a patient's share of healthcare spending, with a maximum annual out-of-pocket expense of $1,000, would lead to reduced "overutilization." The study suggested making patients responsible for 25, 50 or even 95 percent of their individual medical costs through co-insurance, and deductibles. More importantly, Rand concluded that increased patient participation in spending would lead to an overall reduction in spending to only that which funded "appropriate or needed" medical care. Rand's idea was to control a patient's spending behavior to control medical cost and spending. The study gave us a concrete example of the detrimental effect of foregoing the free market system in healthcare, and substituting a centralized, planned market system, and we now know its effects on the delivery of healthcare to patients.

Rand's theory that controlling patient behavior could control spending and prices without suffering consequences is fundamentally flawed. The outcomes have been made more obvious since the launch of ObamaCare. Now we see that patients must pay ever-increasing higher out-of-pocket expenses, yet the price charged for healthcare services continue to spiral out of control.

It is important not to confuse healthcare prices with total healthcare spending. Indeed, from 2007 through 2013, the increase in total healthcare spending slowed considerably, to less than 3.6 percent for 2013. Yet the price of care has not fallen, but continues to move upward. Patients will find the price of health services has increased and as a result, forgo medical treatment because of price. The new

ObamaCare health plans, with their high out-of-pocket limits, do discourage healthcare spending as a growing number of patients are finding themselves in the untenable position of having health insurance, but being unable to afford to use it. They have no resources with which to pay the high deductibles and neither do they have the funds to pay their portion of out-of-pocket expenses each year. Only a tiny number of Americans set aside money to help fund unexpected healthcare expenses.

The ObamaCare mandate exacerbates patient spending decisions by forcing Americans to buy into a funding system that has the power to deny physician-recommended treatment based on what an insurance company deems "inappropriate or unnecessary." Instead of a doctor and patient deciding the best course of care, they both must bend to what insurance actuaries have deemed to be most cost effective for the insurance company. Whether an insurance company is for-profit or non-profit makes no difference when they are the arbiters of care. The fact that federal law places punitive constraints on Americans based on the welfare of private corporate interest – insurance carriers – smacks of cronyism at best, and fascism at worst. Fascism may seem like an extreme term, but consider its tenets; powerful large non-governmental institutions make peace with central government by agreeing to terms that benefit both, at the expense of everyday individuals. Fascism rewards the powerful when they agree to support political leaders in exchange for benefits that give them an advantage over a portion of the economy.

In _America's Bitter Pill_, Steven Brill details the major political influence wielded by the insurance carriers through their national organization, America's Health Insurance Plans (AHIP) as Congressional aides wrote the ObamaCare bill.[12] AHIP, along with a handful of major powerful industry activist groups, designed ObamaCare to benefit their members' interests. AHIP's interest is to maximize insurance premiums and minimize the payment of claims, and to make sure every American is required by law to be covered by a health insurance policy. Giving the insurance carriers additional power to dictate to doctors how to practice medicine, whether directly or indirectly, is an attempt to hold down overall spending through the dictates of a third party, and not based on an individual's medical needs.

A large number of Americans see insurance companies as "The Problem," and therefore support "Medicare for all." Under Medicare for all, every person would be automatically covered for basic healthcare in a government-managed healthcare system such as today's Medicare for seniors. Those who see "Medicare for all" as the panacea to cure U.S. healthcare demonstrate that they know nothing about how damaging the heavy hand of government has been to the delivery of quality healthcare – or they simply don't care. All too often those who back "Medicare for all" do it for political purposes, to win votes.

On the other hand, those who think ObamaCare is the advent of socialized medicine need to look closely at Medicare. Congress passed Medicare in 1965. Its avowed purpose is to ensure that

---

[12] See note 6.

Americans 65 and older will have access to high quality, adequate healthcare. It serves another, darker purpose as it provides socialized, federally-controlled medicine for senior citizens. Like ObamaCare, bureaucrats, politicians, and special interests crafted the Medicare law, and as they wrote it, ignored seeking the advice of patients or doctors who were engaged in medical practice.

Under the guise of beneficence, Medicare forces every working American to pay into its trust fund with the promise that someday in the future, each American will benefit. Medicare needs doctors to fulfil its mission, and conscripts them to provide medical care, paying below-market rates for professional services. Since Medicare's inception, it has become bloated and wasteful, and is subject to tens of billions of dollars each year in fraudulent claims. To add insult to injury seniors who wish to opt out of Medicare must also forego their Social Security benefits locking them into the system against their will. Medicare has succeeded in promoting the concentration of money and power into the hands of favored players such as hospitals and insurance companies, at the expense of physicians and patients.

Examining how medical care is delivered shows the ill effects of Medicare. Consider:

> 1) The use of the Diagnosis Related Group (DRG) to determine how much Medicare will pay a hospital for treating a patient with a particular disease. The level of allowed payment affects the length of time a Medicare patient can stay in the hospital. The hospital's decision to release a Medicare

patient is driven by dollars, not a necessary level of medical care.

2) Congress created the Medicare Payment Advisory Committee (MedPAC) in 1997. MedPAC was charged with advising Congress on how much should be paid to doctors and hospitals for services provided to Medicare patients. Under ObamaCare, MedPAC morphed into the Independent Payment Advisory Board (IPAB) – a board of 15 unelected members appointed by the President. The new law gives IPAB the power to independently set Medicare payments based on its view of how to control overall spending. Overall spending is not determined by a careful analysis of individual cases and medical needs, but by a global approach to budgeting. Global healthcare budgeting when done by governments is, by definition, socialized medicine. IPAB is also charged with approving coverage guidelines and ties the hands of elected members of Congress by making its overrule of IPAB possible only by a supermajority vote.

The IPAB is essentially a healthcare rationing board. Younger people should take no solace thinking this only applies to Medicare (older people). Inevitably, IPAB eventually affects all individuals covered under Medicaid (or other government-paid healthcare) and by extension, will affect private insurance. Remember these two certainties: Private insurers routinely adopt Medicare guidelines for coverage and payment. And, live long enough and you will be covered by Medicare, too.

Doctors and patients need to take a stand now, before these Oba-maCare changes are too deeply engrained. Critical changes to the ACA are needed. Accepting the status quo and the inevitable evolution toward complete socialization of healthcare, will result in patients and physicians being forced into a system that strips away patient privacy and choice while forcing doctors to practice collectivist medicine, sacrificing individualized patient care.

An unacceptable effect of the Affordable Care Act is that it forces doctors to discard their sacred Hippocratic Oath to do no harm. It happens as doctors continue to serve the interests of a government that mandates cost control as more important than an individual's right to determine the course of their own healthcare. Doctors need to quit participating in the immoral system created by Medicare and fueled by the ACA.

According to a Physicians' Foundation study published by Merritt-Hawkins in 2014, more than six percent of physicians today are considering switching to a cash or concierge medical practice where they disavow health insurance contracts and drop out of Medicare and Medicaid and, instead, deal directly with patients on a cash basis.[13] Six percent seems like a small rate, but it represents nearly 50,000 physicians and is a significant indicator of how seriously doctors see their current dilemma.

It is important to recognize that ObamaCare will not work without doctors and patients. Instead of depending on Congress to repeal

[13] See note 7.

ObamaCare, doctors and patients need to work together to repeal it by their actions -- and inactions. Yet, because of the ACA mandate, Americans will be forced to pay for a system that will increase costs for patients, remove healthcare decisions from both the doctor and the patient, and lead to rationing. The ACA will change healthcare as we have known it, as a system based on individual needs, into a system based on one-size-fits-all medicine. This new era of medicine will be cost-controlled, conveyor-belt, socialized medicine.

The surest way to be delivered from ObamaCare is to refuse to participate
.

Dr. Curtis W. Caine summed up the argument for non-participation in a system that is unsustainable economically, and is both morally and ethically bankrupt. These are some steps that doctors and patients can take to regain their freedom:

1. *Physicians can stop participating in Medicaid and Medicare.* Medicare/Medicaid guidelines treat doctors as guilty until proven innocent, accusing them of committing fraud, fomenting waste, and abusing their doctor-patient relationship (a felony). Especially chilling and heinous are government-sanctioned recovery audits which claw back money for services already rendered. Doctors cannot effectively practice good medicine with federal health "police" always looking over their shoulder. To be rid of this onerous

government oversight means dropping out of Medicare and Medicaid programs.

2. *Physicians who plan to stop participating should initiate conversations with their patients about why they have chosen to put patient care above all else.* It is vital that patients understand what we all have at stake in this battle for medical freedom.

3. *Medicare patients whose physicians will no longer participate should have a conversation about costs.* Many physicians are willing to significantly discount services when working directly with patients. It is possible to get more necessary care at less cost.

4. *Patients who have insurance with high deductibles and co-insurances should consider foregoing their insurance for routine visits and tests and go to independent physicians that offer fee-for-service direct pay practices.* These doctors are likely to offer services at discounted prices. In addition, using non-hospital based labs, surgery centers, and radiology facilities can offer significant savings while still delivering high quality care.

5. *If you are healthy, consider getting catastrophic coverage and add supplemental insurance (e.g., accident, critical illness, etc.) or plans such as Aflac.* Most healthy patients see a doctor one or two times a year at an average yearly cost of $400.

Health insurance premiums depend on a variety of factors, including age, where you live, and whether you use tobacco products. Individual annual health insurance premiums may range from $1, 200 a year to several thousands of dollars a year. Family policies often cost more than $15,000 a year, and in some areas of the country, more than $25,000. Almost universally, insurance companies are projecting premium increases – many of double digits – during the next few years.

Besides premiums, health insurance policies often require individuals to pay out-of-pocket expenses in excess of thousands of dollars before the insurance kicks in. It may be more advantageous – if not necessary – to buy a lower premium/high deductible insurance policy and set aside money each month in a Health Savings Account. Deposits made to HSAs, up to a limit, are fully tax deductible. If, for example, you could save $300 a month on premium for a family policy and deposit it into an HSA, your family would have $3,600 to spend on healthcare needs any way you wanted without the risk of denials.

6. *If you are ill, but can't get into a doctor, and have a non-life threatening problem, consider going to an urgent care center*. Get to know the location and reputation of the urgent care centers in your area. Many independent facilities are now staffed by

Board Certified Emergency Room trained physicians and offer excellent care at a fraction of the price of going to a hospital based ER. And you are likely to experience a significantly shorter waiting time when compared to the wait times in an ER.

The United States healthcare system needs many reforms, but the Affordable Care Act is not the solution. Instead of depending on Congress and waiting for each election to bring change, or relying on the U.S. Supreme Court to rule intelligently, it is up to both doctors and patients to work together to take back their power. Taking back patient and physician power will happen as an increasing number of physicians drop out of the third party payer system, and as patients once again embrace their right to control their own medical care. Without a citizen uprising against provisions of the ACA, by their decision, the U.S. Supreme Court and the federal Congress have effectively ended patient-centered medical care.

Chapter 14
The Administration's Answer
to High Healthcare Costs is....
Rationing

"Eternal vigilance is the price of Liberty."
> – Ascribed to several of America's Founding Fathers.

President Obama had much to say about the Affordable Care Act, before, during, and after its passage – he still does. His most infamous and ultimately discredited promises were that an individual could keep their health plan and doctor, and that a family's premiums would be reduced by $2,500 a year. Not only have these statements been shown to be wrong in effect, but journalists have shown they never were true, only political posturing. Given our experience with President Obama's promises, those of his party's Congressional leaders, and the results which can now be evaluated in the light of day, it is increasingly difficult to believe much of what has come out their mouths.

Repeatedly, for instance, President Obama denied his critics who said that his reform would involve rationing of healthcare for those who are the most vulnerable, the senior citizens who depend on Medicare. As ObamaCare emerged from Congress, however, we learned the overall strategy guiding the president's actual proposal to decrease healthcare spending. Guess what? It was rationing. No matter the eventual outcome of this legislation, by passing it the President and Democratic Congressional leaders tipped their hands as how they believed healthcare spending should be controlled.

Section 3403 of the "Patient Protection and Affordable Care Act" established an "Independent [Medicare] Payment Advisory Board." We came to know it as IPAB. These paragraphs from Sec. 3402 define the IPAB's duties:

> "SEC. 1899A. (a) ESTABLISHMENT.—There is established an independent board to be known as the 'Independent [Medicare] Advisory Board'. [Note: Later in the section the word "Medicare" was removed, indicating the IPAB would have broader powers beyond Medicare.]
>
> "(b) PURPOSE.—It is the purpose of this section to, in accordance with the following provisions of this section, reduce the per capita rate of growth in Medicare spending—
>
> "(1) by requiring the Chief Actuary of the Centers for Medicare & Medicaid Services to determine in each year to which this section applies (in this section referred to as 'a determination year') the projected per capita growth rate under Medicare for the second year

following the determination year (in this section referred to as 'an implementation year');

"(2) if the projection for the implementation year ex-
ceeds the target growth rate for that year, *by requiring
the Board to develop and submit during the first year
following the determination year (in this section referred to as 'a proposal year') a proposal containing
recommendations to reduce the Medicare per capita
growth rate to the extent required by this section* [em-
phasis added]; and

"(3) by requiring the Secretary to implement such
proposals unless Congress enacts legislation pursuant
to this section."[14]

The law authorized the president to make the ultimate decision
about whom to appoint to the panel. Once the president chooses the
15 members they must also be confirmed by the U.S. Senate.
Amazingly, the law has no requirement that IPAB members be
practicing physicians, which is a recipe for spending cuts that are
highly likely to negatively affect the delivery of quality individualized patient care.

There are at least two provisions of the law that make it highly unlikely that the IPAB's members would be truly independent. Under
his previously-passed deficit reduction plan, the president proposed
to expand the IPAB's power to increase the GDP growth per capita

---

[14] 111th Congress of the United States of America. (2010) PPACA & HCERA; Public
Laws 111-148 & 111-153: Consolidated Print. Washington, DC. P 387.

cut from the current one percent to five percent. In addition, under his proposal, the IPAB would tightly control Medicaid payments to states and limit access to drugs by controlling spending on prescriptions resulting in the rationing of care.

The IPAB's primary goal ostensibly is to reduce overall spending while maintaining a high quality of care. Two realities, however, doom this idea:

1.   It does nothing to change the exemptions that were given to hospitals and other Medicare providers that make up a majority of Medicare spending, thereby protecting them from the reach of the IPAB.

2.   It will further decrease the already below market rate of Medicare reimbursements to doctors making it even more difficult to provide both quality care for the Medicare patient and to keep their practices open.

The IPAB's effect on access to healthcare should be the overriding factor in evaluating the purpose and potential outcomes of its oversight. If IPABs' goal is to limit healthcare costs by reducing access to physicians, restricting choice of treatments, restricting access to medication and technology, and/or hoping that people will either be too sick or frustrated to access the system while playing the crony politics of rewarding those who helped craft ObamaCare, then it is well on its way to success.

On the other hand, maybe the IPAB can be evaluated on a different basis; if it ever becomes reality.

Remarkably, as of April 2015, the president had not yet appointed anyone to the IPAB and it is unlikely Mr. Obama will ever get the chance. A public outcry erupted over the potential damage the IPAB would do in carrying out its draconian dictates required to cut spending. Former Alaska Governor Sarah Palin set off a firestorm of protest when she infamously labeled the IPAB a "death panel," meaning that in effect, it would begin to choose who would live or die based on how it allowed healthcare dollars to be rationed. Despite the liberal media's outcries against the IPAB's critics, the peoples' mistrust – and two subsequent elections – created great enough pressure on Congress that it has so far, prohibited the president from appointing the IPAB.

After the 2012 election, Congress refused to submit names to President Obama as potential appointees to the IPAB as required by law. In a letter dated May 9, 2013, Republican leaders Speaker of the House John Boehner and Senate Minority Leader Mitch McConnell, wrote to the president:

> Because the law will give IPAB's 15 unelected, unaccountable individuals the ability to deny seniors access to innovative care, we respectfully decline to recommend appointments...
>
> ...your recent budget called for expanding the IPAB by tasking it with making even larger cuts to Medicare

than those called for in the health law, even though the trustees of the Medicare program have told us that IPAB's provider cuts would be "difficult to achieve in practice," because of the denied care that seniors would experience.[15]

John D. Shatto, the Director of the Medicare and Medicaid Cost Estimates Group in the Office of the Actuary at the Centers for Medicare and Medicaid Services (CMS), stated that without the IPAB in place, these duties fall back on the Secretary of Health and Human Services.[16] This suggests that despite the absence of a functioning IPAB, the potential damage it could have done is still in play, and will remain so unless and until Congress repeals the provision.

America's founding fathers knew that liberty can only be preserved by people who pay attention and take action. The public outcry against the IPAB has preserved a degree of liberty and protected our lives, at least for a time, and is a testimony to what can happen when citizens are informed and agitated enough to take action.

[15] Boehner, J.; McConnell, M. (2103). Letter to President Barack Obama, May 6, 2013. Washington, DC.
[16] The editor of this book talked with Mr. Shatto by phone on April 6, 2015, at 11 AM, CDT. Mr. Shatto explained that the president has never appointed the IPAB, and stated the fall back is to place its duties on the Secretary of Health and Human Services.

Chapter 15
ObamaCare = Corporate
Driven Medical Serfdom

If elections tell us anything it's that there are still millions of Americans who believe that ObamaCare will lead us to the healthcare land of milk and honey. It's time to grow up and realize it's never going to happen. We all need to stop and apply an ounce of critical thinking to what Congress has created.

Let's start with this simple consideration: There is no way to enroll 30 million more people into a healthcare system and expect they will have access to care in the manner to which we have become accustomed. Likewise, individuals who have historically carried health insurance must be concerned when 30 million more people flood the system without adding tens of thousands of new doctors to serve them. After all, ObamaCare did not add tens of thousands of doctors or hundreds of clinics to the system. On the contrary, ObamaCare has sent a message to thousands of physicians that they might be wise to consider retiring early.

ObamaCare's proponents employed many arguments to sell the new law to the public, much of it disingenuous. Politicians, activists, unions, and large corporations sold us this law. For the most part doctors on the front line taking care of patients had no voice, and neither were they consulted. As doctors focused on practicing medicine to the best of their ability, corporate interests stepped up, and why not? They stood to gain from new profits gleaned from the practice of corporate disease-driven medicine.

Evidence abounds about who sat "at the table" as Congressional and administrative staff wrote the ObamaCare law. The largest healthcare corporate interests in the country were fighting for their portion of the healthcare dollar. To know who most heavily influenced the partisan policy wonks who wrote the law, examine widespread support from the pharmaceutical industry, the American Medical Association, AARP, The Hospital Corporation of America, America's Health Insurance Plans and their allied associations in the health insurance agent community, and Big Unions.

During the run-up to the passage of ObamaCare, and for months afterward, President Barack Obama, Speaker of the House Nancy Pelosi, and Senate Majority Leader Harry Reid bedazzled Americans with scores of promises. It became confusing to try to navigate through all their claims. These are just a few of the promises they made, but have already been broken:

Myth#1: There is no need to worry about access to primary care doctors.

Fact: The reality is that even before Congress passed the law, there were neither enough primary care doctors nor specialists to take care of the people already in the system. This has been happening in rural areas for years. Now these shortages have become a reality in some large cities. The alphabet soup of regulations such as HIPAA and OSHA, along with the threat of ObamaCare looming on the horizon, have forced private medical practitioners to leave medicine, join larger medical groups, or become hospital employees. Each government action has had the effect of decreasing individual access to timely healthcare services. As a result of a growing difficulty accessing primary care doctors, patients are more likely to have no choice but to seek care from emergency rooms. This trend has continued unabated since the implementation of ObamaCare.

Myth #2: If you like your doctor you can keep him or her.

Fact: Because of the growing dearth of medical doctors, front line providers have already changed. Clinics and hospitals have begun outsourcing healthcare to other, less trained types of healthcare professionals, such as nurse practitioners, physician assistants, and foreign trained doctors. Today, individuals who are lucky enough to see an experienced American-trained doctor find their time together in the exam room to be very short. If ObamaCare is fully implemented and 30 million additional people actually enter the system, the patient's time spent with a full-fledged medical doctor will become rarer.

Myth #3: You will get cheaper, better medical service.

Fact: Overall, ObamaCare has caused healthcare quality to suffer as small-practice intimate care provided by a doctor whom you know is increasingly dominated by large, institutional care. Larger hospitals are buying out smaller community hospitals and hiring doctors who leave their private practices behind. Next, the larger hospitals have joined together to become even-larger specialty centers. Smaller, more cost effective high quality surgery centers are being put out of business, unable to compete with larger hospitals. Small and medium-sized clinics are being merged with ever-larger clinics, and the autonomy of the physicians who work for them is subject to the decision of administrators who keep an eye on the bottom line. This new paradigm is highly regulated by the federal government, on top of state government regulation. As a result of complexity and cost, only Big Medicine has the resources to provide the support necessary to keep up with Big Government. All this eventually means reduced competition resulting in only the most expensive choices for healthcare.

Myth #4: The insurance companies will be brought to heel, no longer able to deny coverage for pre-existing conditions.

Fact: Insurance premiums and profits across the country are soaring. There are many reasons for this. Premiums have increased in part because adult children are allowed to remain on their parents' insurance policies until age 26. This stole away a large number of healthy young people from the insurance medical risk pools, increasing the financial risk for the insurance companies, and thereby the cost of premiums for everyone else.

ObamaCare includes a battery of mandated coverages, many of which are classified as "preventive" care. One of those, requiring insurance companies to pay for birth control, has become the subject of litigation and heated public debate. Yet the birth control mandate, from a standpoint of cost, is tiny compared with the comprehensive cost added by the rest of the mandated preventive care services. The mandates will inevitably raise the premium rates for everyone as insurance companies recoup their increased costs. While premiums increase, so do deductibles and co-insurances. On top of more costly premiums, individuals are paying thousands more out of their own pockets for medical care.

Under ObamaCare, insurance companies cannot deny enrolling people who have pre-existing medical conditions. Much is made of this "no pre-ex" provision, but far too little has been made of the incredible cost it added to insurance premiums. This is another reason why millions of people have found their new ObamaCare premiums to be exorbitant.

Another increased expense comes in the loss of access to medical services as a result of narrower provider networks. If an individual wants to keep his or her doctor, but that doctor is "out of network," the patient is faced with a choice: He or she can stay in the network but lose access to their preferred physician, or can leave the network, but pay far more for care. Insurance companies insist that ObamaCare forced them to negotiate these new narrower networks in order to restrain premium growth (one can only imagine the upward spike in rates if everyone could go to whichever doctor they preferred).

Insurance companies, as well, have adopted more hurdles to care in the name of holding down spending. One of the strategies they use is requiring pre-certification of services. If a doctor believes a specific test is necessary, he or she might first have to get approval from the insurance carrier. This pre-certification requirement serves to delay or deny medical services. The other strategy adopted by insurance companies has been to limit covered prescriptions allowed in their formulary shifting the increasing cost to patients.

Myth #5: Electronic Medical Records (EMR) will improve care by allowing your health information to be more easily accessed by other healthcare professionals.

Fact: EMR purveyors sell the idea of "interoperable" digital records as a way for all medical professionals to see your personal history, avoid mistakes, cut down on diagnosis time, and produce better outcomes. EMRs, however, come with a heavy cost. They have added another layer of administrative expense for doctors and hospitals, and they must pass that cost on to individuals through higher insurance premiums and charges for medical services.

The noble goal of making your personal medical records available in real-time to anyone who provides medical services to you requires sophistication not yet available anywhere in the world. It requires being able to digitally tie together your personal records with tens of millions of others, all generated through billions of transactions every day, and allow access to yours only among all the others. It assumes that all systems will be able to talk to each other, without error. Whether this can ever be achieved is unknown, but what is known is that we are far from it.

There are other risks to consider.

EMRs are not only shared among healthcare professionals, but also with the Department of Health and Human Services and myriad other government agencies.

1. Digital record-sharing has the potential to have a chilling effect on the doctor patient relationship. When personal information that is protected by health information privacy is shared with the Secretary of Health and Human Services, it leaves the patient and physician vulnerable. There is the potential for the patient to have his or her personal information used against them (for example if they try to seek government employment or contracts) in a variety of settings. With the interplay of the Internal Revenue Service serving as the financial watchdog over individual health insurance enrollment, the potential for foul play is heightened.

2. EMRs weaken the safety of personal information and make it more vulnerable to a potential breach from hacking. This leaves patients and doctors vulnerable to financial attack, and gives others the potential to use private information to extort and defraud individuals.

3. Sharing all this patient data with bureaucrats puts the government in the powerful position of looking over the doc-

tor's shoulder. Government agencies can penalize physicians who, compelled to practice the "art" of care, perform procedures outside of the strict treatment guidelines upon which ObamaCare's mandated one-size-fits-all medical care (aka Evidence Based Medicine) is based.

EMRs seem to be the perfect model for a centralized healthcare system that seeks to control spending, make decisions on behalf of individual patients and doctors, and brings everyone into conformity. ObamaCare's proponents sold us this new law as the cure-all for our ailing healthcare system. Now that we've read the bill, it's become apparent that it has never been about medicine – it is about control.

CHAPTER 16
BOXING, WRESTLING, AND NOW
THE AFFORDABLE CARE ACT:
IS THE FIX IN?

When, on June 28, 2012, I sat listening to news reports about the Supreme Court's <u>NFIB v. Sebelius</u> decision my mood changed from hopeful euphoria to utter disbelief. The last time I had felt this way was while watching the Manny Pacquiao fight against Timothy Bradley on June 9, 2012. Pacquiao won, in my view and the view of thousands who watched the fight, but the judges saw it otherwise. On June 21, after reviewing the fight, the WBO Championship Committee judges declared that indeed, Pacquiao should have won – but they could not change the outcome.

In NFIB v. Sebelius, court-watchers from all stripes thought for sure that the Roberts' Court would overturn the ACA's individual mandate to buy insurance as unconstitutional. Like those of us who were certain Pacquiao had won, it seemed like June 28, 2012 would breathe new life into the health reform movement. Instead, the court upheld the ACA on the basis that Congress has the constitutional power to levy taxes. Like the Pacquiao/Bradley judges who refused to believe their own eyes, the SCOTUS apparently failed to actually read the bill that created the new law. The bill says nothing about the requirement to purchase insurance as a tax, but instead, labeled it "Individual Responsibility," calling it a "Requirement to maintain minimum essential coverage."[17] Everyone who read it, and the media that reported on it, knew it meant that the new law forced individuals to purchase health insurance or enroll in a government health plan. Everyone knew, too, that it was not a tax. ObamaCare's advocates swore that the tenets of the bill were not based on taxing Americans – the SCOTUS ruled that was a lie.

Once the Court announced its NFIB ruling, we knew that like it or not, we would have to contend with the law's effects. We quickly began to learn many of the details of the ACA disease that will ultimately kill the American system of healthcare. The ACA's effects are to destroy the doctor-patient relationship on the one hand and eliminate both the doctors' freedom to treat, and patients' freedom to choose treatment options on the other hand.

The bill passed with all Democratic votes, the political party that purports to be the champion of the American middle class and working poor. Instead of championing them, the Democrats had crafted and passed a law that has saddled those very people with the largest tax hike this country has ever seen. Americans seemed to have caught on to their lie, and in three election cycles thereafter, culminating in 2014, elected a Republican majority to both the U.S. House and Senate.

---

[17] 111th Congress. Patient Protection and Affordable Care Act – Consolidated print. Page. 2 and Page 136ff. Washington, DC. January 5, 2010.

Americans who viewed, or continue to view the ACA as their door to good healthcare are in for a rude awakening – starting with increased taxes, since everyone will pay them in one way or another. Americans for Tax Reform (ATR) highlighted 20 new or higher taxes that will affect American families and small businesses.[18] ATR published the following list after examining provisions in the ACA, provisions that directly affect the quality, access, and/or price of healthcare and are sure to negatively impact the American people:

Tax on Innovator Drug Companies ($22.2 billion – Effective Jan 2010): $2.3 billion annual tax on the industry imposed relative to share of sales made that year. This will likely affect patient access to innovative treatments because the cost of creating new medications will increase.

Medicine Cabinet Tax ($5 billion – Effective Jan 2011): Americans no longer are able to use Health Savings Account (HSA), Flexible Spending Account (FSA), or Health Reimbursement Arrangements (HRA) pre-tax dollars to purchase non-prescription, over-the-counter medicines (except insulin). This is simply a gift to the pharmaceutical industry since it influences a decision to save money, while increasing access to the most expensive option. This is exacerbated by the inability for Americans to freely import drugs at a reduced price.

[18] http://www.atr.org/tax-hikes-obamaCare-scotus-rule-a6996

Hike in Medicare Payroll Tax ($86.8 billion – Effective Jan 2013): Translated: more taxes on middle income families.

Raise "Haircut" for Medical Itemized Deduction from 7.5 percent of Adjusted Gross Income (AGI) to 10 percent of AGI ($15.2 billion – Effective Jan 2013): Prior to 2013, those facing high medical expenses were allowed a deduction for medical spending to the extent that those expenses exceed 7.5 percent of adjusted gross income (AGI). The new provision imposes a threshold of 10 percent of AGI. (Waived for 65+ taxpayers in 2013-2016 only.) This will increase the net cost of healthcare for individuals who lose the previous tax deduction, or who now must meet the higher threshold before being able to deduct their medical spending.

Elimination of tax deduction for employer-provided retirement Rx drug coverage in coordination with Medicare Part D ($4.5 billion – Effective Jan 2013) This negates the "closing of the donut hole" and raises costs for seniors.

Excise Tax on Comprehensive Health Insurance Plans ($32 billion – Effective Jan 2018): Starting in 2018, new 40 percent excise tax on "Cadillac" health insurance plans ($10,200 single/$27,500 family). Higher threshold ($11,500 single/$29,450 family) for early retirees and high-risk professions. CPI +1 percentage point indexed. This affects most PPO plans (the ones that give patients the most freedom to choose their doctor – they generally also have less out of pocket expenses for patients.) This will effectively relegate people to HMO types of plans with the least choice in doctors, higher out of pocket expenses and gatekeepers that require patients to have referrals to see specialists.

NOTE: As the deadline for the Cadillac tax approached, savvy healthcare finance professionals realized something; it should be called the Chevy tax, or maybe even the Kia tax because they will affect middle class Americans. Given the premium spikes generated by over-rich ObamaCare health plans, the ones mandated by the ACA and the regulations it spun off, millions of wealthy and middle class policyholders will find themselves subject to the 40 percent assessment. This will be especially true if they benefit from Health Reimbursement Arrangements (HRA), Health Savings Accounts (HSA) or have Flexible Spending Accounts (FSA). All of the funds paid for premium and these other arrangements will be used to tally up the total value of a health plan, and hence, usher in the Cadillac/Chevy tax on everyday Americans.

It took until late in 2014 before nearly all insurance agents discovered yet another tax boost, this one determined by ACA regulations on employer provided health insurance. Many policymakers had hoped the ACA would encourage a rapid increase in the number of employees who choose an individual health insurance policy over enrolling in an employer's plan. Yet, the ACA-regulators read the new law in such a way as to deny any tax preference to those individuals. Instead of receiving a health insurance benefit from their employers, under the new regulations, any money paid to employees in lieu of the health insurance benefit is considered employee income and therefore subject to the full array of federal and state taxes. This means that employees, forced to enroll in expensive ObamaCare insurance plans, will also see their taxes go up. These increased taxes, paradoxically, directly or indirectly subsidize health insurance for other people.

ObamaCare's proponents sold it to Americans using smoke and mirrors. Professor Jonathan Gruber, the mastermind behind Massachusetts' healthcare reform, and who later played a central role in creating ObamaCare, admitted this in a candid moment when he said the American people are stupid. Gruber went on to say that if the American people (read voters) knew the details of ObamaCare they never would have supported it. In 2009, in a public policy paper he openly explained that "ObamaCare had no cost controls and would not be affordable."

> "The problem is it starts to go hand in hand with the mandate; you can't mandate insurance that's not affordable. This is going to be a major issue," Gruber admitted in an October 2, 2009 lecture...
>
> "So what's different this time? Why are we closer than we've ever been before? Because there are no cost controls in these proposals. Because this bill's about coverage. Which is good! Why should we hold 48 mil-

lion uninsured people hostage to the fact that we don't yet know how to control costs in a politically accept-able way? Let's get the people covered and then let's do cost control."

Gruber also said that the only way to control costs is to effectively deny treatment.

"The real substance of cost control is all about a sin-gle thing: telling patients they can't have something they want. It's about telling patients, 'That surgery doesn't do any good, so if you want it you have to pay the full cost.'"[19]

Jonathan Gruber played a central role in creating and rolling out the Massachusetts Connector. Massachusetts, therefore, provides us with a glimpse into our future. Massachusetts' healthcare costs have risen since its General Court (state legislature) created its state insurance exchange in 2006. At the start, people gamed the system carrying coverage when they became ill, and dropping it when they recovered. Pundits labeled these people "jumpers" and "dumpers." Eventually, the Massachusetts' legislature created a once-per-year open enrollment period and ObamaCare's authors carried that idea forward into the new federal law.

The passage of RomneyCare (as some call it) has created other sys-temic problems. For instance, wait times to see a doctor have in-

[29] Howley, P. (2014) Obama Advisor Jonathan Gruber In 2009: ObamaCare will NOT Be Affordable. The Daily Caller. Retrieved 4/8/2015. http://dailycaller.com/2014/12/30/obama-adviser-jonathan-gruber-in-2009-obamaCare-will-not-be-affordable/

creased. Scheduling an appointment with a new primary care doctor can stretch out to more than 60 days. As reimbursements to physicians and hospitals fell some doctors fled the state and others refused to see new patients. Consistently, some 85 percent of enrollees through the Massachusetts' exchange receive government subsidies yet physicians are reluctant to care for them at a financial loss. The net result? Massachusetts residents have seen a reduction in access to quality care, but at higher prices and increased taxes.

When the Supreme Court relied on Congress' power to tax in deciding NFIB v. Sebelius, it set up Americans for a fundamental change. Since it creates a system which has the potential to destroy the American dream of a thriving middle class by transferring wealth from the 99 percent to those at the top who control the healthcare dollars. The question remains is it one that Americans can believe in?

Americans should rise up against this redistribution of wealth and loss of liberty. Doctors and their patients must stop playing the ACA game and instead, move to a free market system that removes the corporate and government middle men. The answer lies in going back to the basics. Patients and doctors need to re-enter a fee-for-service system featuring pricing transparency, re-learn how to personally pay for routine medical care, and purchase catastrophic insurance for major medical and hospital expenses.

One of the clearest indicators that Congress' and President Obama's true intent is to federalize healthcare and reduce patient freedom is the ACA's assault on Consumer Directed Healthcare. This bias against consumerism is easily observed by listening to healthcare bureaucrats at all levels blame fee-for-service medicine as evil and in its place, praising highly structured, top-down managed care as holy and pure. Big Medicine prefers Accountable Care Organizations, evidence-based practice guidelines, IPAB, and the almost unending number of federal healthcare officers, over the doctor-patient relationship which is based on face-to-face, one-on-one medicine. Whereas in a consumerized system, the patient must know the price of medical care, in the new ACA world, the price is known only to contract managers and their counterparts at the insurance companies and in the federal government. Instead of paying $75 to see a doctor, the patient now pays $750 in monthly premium into a system that sucks most of the money out of it and then pays thousands of dollars in taxes to support others' who need help paying their unaffordable premiums while artificially putting a value on care given by physicians. Welcome to the new logic of the ACA's tax and spend system of medicine.

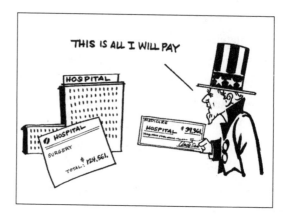

CHAPTER 17
A BRIEF PRIMER ON REIMBURSEMENTS

The next chapter will discuss how physician and hospital "reimbursements" rely on a complicated coding system. Before moving on, however, we offer a brief primer on the reimbursement system that should prove helpful.

Nearly all medical care in the United States is provided through a reimbursement system that accomplishes several purposes. First, it is a way to pay professionals for the services they provide. Second, since almost all reimbursements flow through third party payers, reimbursements give the payers a significant level of control over the practice of medical professionals. If a professional wishes to be paid for his or her time, it means performing services that are reimbursable and authorized under the payer's contract with the professional.

"Cash practice" doctors have addressed the issue of third party reimbursements and the control it imposes on them by refusing third party reimbursements as a method of payment. In this way, the cash practice physician is able to examine a patient but also discuss the cost required to access a therapy or treatment regimen. Together, the physician and the patient decide what course of care is reasonable and the cost is transparent. There is no need to rely on a Third Party Payer which adds bureaucratic cost to the service while telling them what they can and cannot do.

Under the system of being paid through reimbursements, instead of the patient/client paying for a service at the time they receive it, the "patient" pays later, by "reimbursing" the provider. The physician performs the service and bills the client through the payer. Then the professional waits for a "reimbursement" to be paid. The reimbursement comes from any one or a combination of these: insurance companies, third party administrators, government agencies, or from the patient. When an individual is uninsured or not enrolled in a government health plan, the reimbursement comes directly from the patient. When the patient uses a third party option such as an insurance company, the only portion of the billing for which payment is due at the time of service are co-pays, and these are a fraction of the real cost of care.

Unlike doctors, hospitals, and other medical providers, very few others are paid after-the-fact through a reimbursement program such as that of our healthcare system. Imagine your auto mechanic waiting 60-90 days to be paid by a third party for changing your oil or your plumber waiting to be paid after fixing a leak – it does not happen. Lawyers ask for hefty retainers when they take your case, before lifting a finger, and they are not shy about asking for more money as your case moves along. Try to stop paying your lawyer and watch your case grind to a halt. Tell the clothing store clerk you'll be sure to get a check to the store within 90 days as you walk out the door in your new outfit, and see how far you will get before a mall cop nabs you.

When you walk into a doctor's office, however, you expect to receive all the care you want or need without having to pay the bill before leaving the clinic. Under your health plan you have no idea how much the insurance company will reimburse the doctor for providing care to you. Other than your co-pay, the doctor must wait to be reimbursed for providing medical care to you.

Paying for most healthcare, especially emergency care or treatments that require major expense, is different from most other services, and it often needs to be. There are instances when requiring payment on the spot for medical care is inappropriate, and the reimbursement system does allow for a method of managing those costs over time. Imagine laying on a gurney in an emergency room, having suffered a heart attack, but being denied care until you can write a check. This does not usually happen in our U.S. healthcare finance system,[20] although true enough, there is an intake nurse meeting with your next of kin, taking down insurance information while the ER physician is examining you. The difference is that no one is going to ask you to pay before emergency care is provided. If you are uninsured, what happens after the care is provided can get contentious, but we generally do not deny care to people in these situations. The hospital in which the ER is located or the Ur-

---

[20] Occasionally we hear of over-aggressive collection companies trying to secure payment from a patient in an Emergency Room. This is not the normal practice of most emergency departments.

gent Care Center where the patient may have gone first will have to wait for reimbursement.

It would be helpful if we could change the way we talk about payments for medical care. Instead of talking about "how the doctor gets reimbursed," we should say "how the doctor gets paid." In fact, thousands of doctors have severed their ties to the reimbursement system and now get paid directly by patients at the time when the services are provided.

The reimbursement system of payment requires an extraordinary amount of complicated record-keeping. It also plays well for those who believe in a top-down healthcare management system that inserts itself between the doctor and patient. As normally practiced today, it is a perverse adaptation of the Golden Rule. In this case, "He who has the gold makes the rules." If the payment comes from a third party payer, then the rules come from the bureaucracy. If the payment comes from the patient, then the patient rules and the physicians love it.

Chapter 18
Being Pro-Healthcare Reform and Against ObamaCare

It is important to clarify a key contention between those who support ObamaCare and those who oppose it. ObamaCare proponents are quick to say that those that oppose the ACA are against healthcare reform. By implication, if you are an ObamaCare detractor then you are also accused of trying to maintain the status quo, or protect Big Medicine, or selfishly protecting your own turf while ignoring the welfare of others. The truth, however, is far different.

Prior to Congress' passing the ACA, widespread agreement existed across the country that the United States healthcare system needed reform, or as author Dave Racer insists, "healthcare redesign."[21] Physicians have continuously been in favor of redesigning our ways of delivering and paying for medical care and are, in fact, active participants in doing so, if allowed. Congress has been redesigning healthcare by legislative fiat for more than 75 years, and each time it does, it seems as though we move farther away from a patient-physician centered system and instead, expand bureaucratic oversight and cost.

[21] Racer, D. (2010) *Comprehensive Healthcare Redesign: 25 Keys to Redesign U.S. Healthcare*. Alethos Press. St. Paul, MN. September 2010.

Medical care is, by nature, subject to continuous evaluation and refinement as science, technology, information, pharmacology, and advances in surgery plunge ahead. Physicians are always adapting to changes and most doctors have strong opinions on how to do it better. This is one reason that in the midst of ObamaCare reforms, an increasing number of physicians are opting out of Medicare, Medicaid, CHIP, and other forms of government-reimbursement systems, and severing their contracts with insurance companies. When a physician redesigns his or her practice by providing care on a cash basis, it requires significant changes in how they deliver and are paid for providing medical services.

It is disingenuous to suggest that opposing the Affordable Care Act is the same as opposing healthcare reform. The reality is that many of us want to discard the ACA and create reforms that actually work, and that favor the patient-physician relationship. We are ready to redesign healthcare by starting with dumping the ACA.

The point here is that ObamaCare is far more than "reform," it is a radical makeover of how we deliver and pay for healthcare. It is a federalization of our healthcare system. ObamaCare means entrusting the lives and fortunes of more than 320 million Americans to bureaucrats in Washington, DC, and their corporate partners – that is unhealthy. Millions of Americans and tens of thousands of physicians oppose the federalization of healthcare, but they strongly favor redesigning its processes and payment systems.

CHAPTER 19
COOKBOOK HEALTHCARE:
THE FUTURE OF MEDICINE IN
THE UNITED STATES

Have you wondered how the 2010 healthcare reform law – The Affordable Care Act – will play out over time in the United States? To best understand this, one needs only to look at how the World Health Organization (WHO) has designed it.

The International Classification of Disease (ICD) code system is an emerging powerhouse in the provision of and payment for healthcare. WHO uses ICD codes to classify diseases. Third party payers also use ICD codes as the basis for reimbursements to hospitals and physicians. The physician who is under contract to insurance companies and the various government health plans have no choice but to use ICD codes in order to be paid.

The ICD codes have gone through numerous revisions and expansions. The most recent is titled ICD-10. As of this writing, 25 countries have adopted it.[22] The Czech Republic adopted it in 1994.

---

[22] ICD-10. http://en.wikipedia.org/wiki/ICD-10#National_adoption_for_clinical_use Retrieved on 1/6/2015

Australia, in 1998; then Canada in 2000. The most recent country to adopt it was Thailand in 2007.

The United States had been scheduled to adopt it in 2013, but like so much related to the ACA, Washington, DC bureaucrats delayed the date. "The deadline for the United States to begin using Clinical Modification ICD-10-CM for diagnosis coding and Procedure Coding System ICD-10-PCS for inpatient hospital procedure coding is [now] set at October 1, 2015..."[23] U.S. implementation of ICD-10 is yet another major piece of the healthcare reform law to take effect.

Congress' mad rush to pass healthcare reform makes a lot of sense when one considers the hoped-for timetable for implementation of ICD-10. If it had not been delayed due to federal bureaucratic interference, the U.S. would already be fully integrated into the global healthcare system overseen by the World Health Organization. Soon enough, unless the law is changed, we will be there.

ACA managers claim that 30 million more individuals will be enrolled in healthcare coverage than were enrolled prior to the ACA. If that happens, in what ways will our healthcare system change when so many millions more seek access to healthcare? Indeed, during April 2015, news reports signaled that healthcare spending has begun to grow more rapidly than in previous years. One reason this growth is occurring, the reports state, is because hospital use has grown, and the growth is attributed to more people having health insurance. It is well-known that once uninsured people gain

[43] Ibid.

health coverage they actually use it. The British Columbia, Canada experience provides an example of what we can expect.

BC uses a series of clinical treatment guidelines set forth by a protocols advisory committee to determine how a physician should practice in any given medical situation. The ACA, likewise, sets up an advisory panel that will use "evidence based medicine" to determine appropriate medical care. These advisory panels design treatment flow sheets that will, it is hoped, make it easy for non-physician healthcare providers – i.e. physician assistants, nurse practitioners – to provide care. Knowing how this plan is expected to work put the comments of former Pennsylvania Governor Ed Rendell into context. Rendell said that healthcare providers, referring to non-physician providers, are "just as good as primary care physicians."

Rendell is not worried about the pending physician shortage because his belief is clearly based on the premise that anyone can use algorithms to provide cookbook medical care. All one needs to do is connect the dots.

In theory, cookbook medicine sounds great, but fails when applied to the real world. Take for example the treatment of middle ear infections or sore throats. I have treated many children whose pediatrician who finally refers them to an ENT specialist after months of recurrent ear infections. Instead of referring the child sooner for ENT evaluation and ventilation tubes, the doctor simply followed practice guidelines set forth by evidence based medicine, until the illness became chronic. After the condition worsens it can affect the child's hearing leading to problems performing in school such as speech delay. By the time the primary care physician refers them to me they have suffered a great deal and their case is far more severe than it would have been if treated early on. I have put ventilation tubes in children who had been placed in special education for a perceived learning disability or ADD when it was simply their inability to hear due to a chronic ear infection. It was immensely gratifying to hear how well the child performed in school or how much their behavior had changed after surgery.

Those professionals charged with designing practice guidelines want to eliminate unnecessary medical procedures to reduce spending for medical care, but they need to take an individual patient into consideration. Minimizing expenditures may be right in some cases, or even in most. All Big Data can do is predict outcomes based on a presumed norm. If the guidelines tell the physician to treat symptoms in a way that is least expensive, it may appear right on the digital spreadsheet, but can actually waste money in the long run. What is lost in these practice guidelines is the common sense fact that in some patients a surgical intervention is cheaper in the long run because it can solve the underlying problem instead of managing the symptom. The decision on the best treatment for each patient is best made by the attending physician, not by a data set stored in a government facility.

As ObamaCare ratchets up its data collection regime it will create an enormous amount of information, and technocratic medical researchers will declare they have found "the" way to treat each symptom. The one-size-fits-all approach to medical care downplays the importance of individualized care. Although those who write the guidelines base them on research – even extensive research – they will inevitably lag behind what patients experience in the real world. Ignoring the real world will have a negative impact on individualized patient care.

For example, the Canadian Advisory Panel guideline for the treatment of sore throats is not true. "With the exception of rare infections by certain pharyngeal bacterial pathogens (e.g., Corynebacterium diphtheriae, Neisseria gonorrhoeae and Arcanobacterium haemolyticum), antimicrobial therapy is of no proven benefit in the treatment of acute pharyngitis due to bacteria other than group A streptococcus." Just before I first wrote this chapter, I had drained an abscess on a patient. The patient's physician, who followed practice guidelines, had not prescribed antibiotics because the strep test had been negative. The patient, however, actually had a staphylococcal infection.

The assumption that a blanket application of Big Data can be applied to all medical cases will reduce the quality of all healthcare. When applied to other diseases, such as screening mammograms and other ailments, practice guidelines can lead to people falling through clinical cracks and getting sicker, ultimately requiring more expensive and invasive care.

This is the single most important "practice guideline:" The practice of good medicine will always be unpredictable and will require physicians to practice medicine as an art, not a computer algorithm. It is the physician who is in the room examining the patient that provides the best practices for that individual at that moment in time.

ICD-10 codes forced upon physicians and then used by Big Data researchers who tell physicians how to practice will stultify innovation and short-circuit physician-patient interaction. Worrying about getting the ICD-10 codes entered correctly to avoid a fine and ensure a reimbursement does not lead to patient-centered care, but this is our future under ObamaCare.

CHAPTER 20
DISENFRANCHISED AND
DUPED BY OBAMACARE

"Seeing is believing," is the adaptation of the words of the Disciple Thomas when he first saw Jesus Christ after His resurrection. Modern politics does its best to hide behind images and rhetoric, not facts. Its outcomes, however, should be judged by what we see, not what we believe or are made to believe by the message manipulators. Based on this evaluation we can say without hesitation – today's political leadership is no longer about the content of one's character, it is all about winning at all costs.

The 2012 re-election of Barack Obama showed how powerful the blind and dogged devotion of Progressives are to ObamaCare is. Despite the ACA's architects' admission that the law is inherently unfair, and the delays, obfuscations, and outright lies voters have witnessed – many from the president's lips – Obama's backers were still able to convince Americans it would all work out as long as they sent him back to the White House. Their ruse worked long enough to get "folks" to the voting booths to vote "Obama."

Those 2012 voters never witnessed an open debate about ObamaCare. If they had, they would have seen how it creates a two-tiered medical system that will, in the long term, benefit the wealthy and privileged, while relegating the poor, middle class, and disenfranchised to inferior healthcare. Medicare enrollees, and those who soon will be enrolled, would have seen how ObamaCare will eventually force them into huge medical systems that are concerned more about how not to spend money on medical care than on caring for those with medical needs. An honest, open debate about ObamaCare would have shown voters how the ACA makes the best quality doctors unavailable to them, and how far too many Americans will be locked out of access to the best quality healthcare at medical centers of excellence like Sloan-Kettering Cancer Center and MD Anderson. In an open and honest election debate, voters would have discovered that very soon, they would be stuck paying higher costs for health insurance, medication, and paying more expenses out-of-pocket. Instead, the political establishment sold ObamaCare as if it is a new right with which no politician should meddle and the complexity of healthcare combined with the media's unwillingness to attempt to explain it, left most people without a clue about what was going on.

"Seeing is believing." The cheerleaders of this ghoulish ACA system apparently think it is okay for people to die from a lack of access due to high insurance or medical care prices, or from denial of medical services deemed to be either medically unnecessary, experimental, or simply too expensive. The statisticians and actuaries distill the real human costs down to numbers, and spin those numbers into talking points designed to sell a political message. The campaign strategists decide the message, because it is more important to be on the winning team no matter the consequences for everyday Americans.

For those Progressives who sincerely believe in this ACA system, it brings a whole new meaning to "taking one for the team." So committed are the ObamaCare sycophants to their system and their president, they will cry "racism" or "discrimination against the sick and the elderly" or a "war against women" any time someone questions their veracity. They kill the debate before it can start. Theirs' is an immoral and unfair approach to political debate because demonizes the opponent in order to shut down debate.

It is past time to demand that Americans really live by Dr. Martin Luther King Jr's call for people to be judged by the content of their character instead of being silenced by hypocritical race hustlers who want to control our destiny. The race card, and now the gender card, has been over-played for too long. Time has come for Americans to get past this and ignore the banal cries of those who want to create and perpetuate victimhood in order to win political power. Instead, we must work to expose their dark deeds, manipulative, focus-group tested words, and the candidates they support – and reject them. It is imperative that we confront this deception because, ever since passage of the ACA, in a very real sense, our lives are at stake.

In 2014, some media sources finally began to report the astonishing words of a chief ObamaCare architect, Jonathan Gruber, PhD. Gruber is a professor at the Massachusetts Institute of Technology, and played a primary role in getting "RomneyCare" passed in Massachusetts in 2006, eventually becoming a member of its insurance exchange board of directors. He took credit for key elements of ObamaCare as it rolled out, and went on the road to sell its virtues. At one point he proclaimed in essence that 20 years from now, everyone would love the new law and tell lawmakers to leave it alone. So when media finally reported on Gruber's proclamation about "the stupidity of the American voter" as a reason Obama could not be transparent and truthful about the law,[24] the truth finally emerged. The ACA's proponents had lied when they sold it to the American people, and continue to do so today.

It will take years before Americans are able to understand the effects of the depth of deception spun by the Obama administration and the members of Congress who gave us ObamaCare. There will never be full disclosure of its effects on withholding or delay of care because it is nearly impossible to document. Very few physicians, especially those who are employed by big health systems, will take the time to step forward and tell what happens in their examination rooms and surgical theaters, and how patients are being disfavored. Worse yet, no doctor will be able to tell the stories of individuals who never came to them. Occasionally, however, a story emerges that indicates the disasters that lay just below the surface of public awareness, but may bubble up from time to time. Such is the story of Charlie Dunker.

[44] Howley, P. (2014) *ObamaCare Architect: Lack of Transparency Was Key Because 'Stupidity of the American Voeter" Would have Killed ObamaCare.* The Daily Caller. Washington, DC. 11/09/2014. Retrieved 4/15/2015.
http://dailycaller.com/2014/11/09/obamacare-architect-lack-of-transparency-was-key-because-stupidity-of-the-american-voter-would-have-killed-obamacare/ (and there are scores of additional sources verifying this same revelation)

On March 16, 2015, Dunker of Jackson, Minnesota appeared before a Minnesota House Committee. He laid out the tragic tale of how the Minnesota health insurance exchange's incompetence cost his wife, Gail Dunker, her life. The Dunker's applied for insurance coverage through MNsure, Minnesota's problem-plagued insurance exchange. MNsure has had a chronic problem of struggling to fix problems on an individual basis. MNsure could never fix the Dunker's situation and Charlie blames the exchange for her death.

> For months, the couple was uninsured as they fought with MNsure to finalize their enrollment, causing problems as they sought tests and appointments, he said.

> "She was in Mayo [Clinic] from November to Jan. 9, when she died," he said, pausing to pull out two photos of his wife, Gail -- one a portrait, and the other of her lying in a hospital bed. "When MNsure was jerking our chain, that's what happened. That's why I'm here."[25]

True to political form, within minutes of telling his heart-wrenching story, Rep. Tina Liebling, D-Rochester, had to offer "balance." Liebling, a single-payer advocate, told how one of her constituents who suffers from depression and substance abuse had enrolled in Medicaid through MNsure and, as a result, received much needed

[25] Montgomery, D. (2015) Kill MNsure? Maybe, Dayton Says. 3/17/2015. The St Paul Pioneer Press. St. Paul MN. Retrieved on 4/16/2015.
http://www.twincities.com/news/ci_27723220/kill-mnsure?-maybe-dayton-says

care. No one argues that some people benefit from government health plans, but everyone, Rep. Liebling's constituent and Gail Dunker, deserve equal consideration from ObamaCare. Dunker never got it, and that is the nature of healthcare – it is an individual proposition to a patient, not a number on a government health plan registration form.

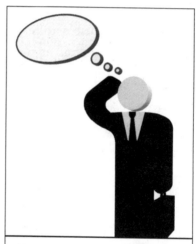

ObamaCare's authors relied on professional academics, researchers, politicians and their staff members, and physicians who were not practicing medicine. They could ask questions, but had little to no understanding of the implications of their answers.

Chapter 21
Six Ways Your Health Insurance Company Makes it Hard for Your Doctor to Take Care of You

Many Americans have a misconception about the reasons health-care prices are so high – and always seemingly going higher. Some lay major blame on an alleged frequency of unnecessary procedures related to doctors' practice of defensive medicine. Defensive medicine is defined as when a doctor provides unnecessary care only to avoid a potential lawsuit, or an angry patient.

The 2014 Merritt-Hawkins survey of physicians found that 51 percent of physicians believe that defensive medicine contributes to rising healthcare costs.[26] It is common for healthcare reformers to point to these statistics and then blame the physicians for doing what is actually quite rational. The reality is that if a physician, who practices in a state with weak malpractice laws, feels as though he or she is always looking over a shoulder to see if a trial attorney lingers nearby, then yes, that physician might be tempted to do more than otherwise might be necessary. Blaming the physician, however, is misguided. This dilemma can best be addressed

---

[26] See note 7.

by fixing the malpractice laws to reduce the number of nuisance lawsuits.

It is popular for the media, along with some politicians and activists, to blame the high cost of care on physician salaries, and especially, on fee-for-service billings. Physicians, however, who are daily engaging in healthcare transactions, see it differently. Only 10.3 percent blame fee-for-service billings and just 2.1 percent blame it on physician fees.[27] Of course, the physicians' response might seem self-serving, but they also understand the nature of the forces behind the pricing of healthcare services, and their fees are not the cause.

In my experience, I have seen how the medical insurance industry has fueled a campaign of misinformation as part of a divide-and-conquer strategy. As long as patients blame doctors, they pay less attention to rising deductibles, co-insurance, out-of-pocket expenses, and escalating premiums. In short, the insurance companies benefit by keeping doctors and patients at odds with each other. In reality, the amount the insurance company pays a doctor or hospital is nowhere near the amount of the original bill. The billing system preferred by insurance companies leaves doctors, hospitals, and patients confused.

Instead of blaming doctors for the price of medical care, those who pay the ever-skyrocketing cost of health insurance should take a closer look at the salaries of health insurance administrators and CEOs.

[27] See note 8.

These are six things you need to know so you can understand the barriers with which your doctor has to navigate to take good care of you:

1. Insurance companies change the procedures for which they will pay.

Using a pre-certification process, insurance companies will change the services for which they will "reimburse" a doctor. The list of procedures for which insurance will pay can change periodically. Whether or not to pay is driven by insurance company costs and not by medical necessity as determined by the doctor and the patient. If the procedure or treatment is covered, the doctor will be paid, but if the insurance company drops the procedure out of its authorized list, the physician will not be paid unless they can persuade the patient to ante up.

2. Insurance companies employ gatekeepers that look for reasons to deny recommended services.

Insurance companies have physicians and/or nurses on their administrative staff that can deny services. The person that reviews a medical service to determine whether it is covered may not even be someone familiar with the medical procedure (for example, a psychiatrist reviewing a surgeon's notes relating to the need for a surgical procedure).

3. Insurance gatekeepers get bonus compensation when they save the company money.

This is self-explanatory – it pays to deny care.

4. Insurance companies discount payments for surgery and other procedures.

This process is called bundling. If a medical procedure has a left and right side like knee surgery, or has several steps, like sinus surgery, the surgeon will be paid a rate steeply discounted from the billed amount that can be as high as 80 percent. For example, a surgeon will be paid the discounted insurance allowed amount for the first side and 50 percent for the second side. If it is a multi-step procedure, the surgeon will be paid the allowed amount for the first step, 50 percent for the second step, and 25 percent for the third through fifth steps, and nothing for anything beyond the fifth step.

5. Insurance companies make a bigger profit by delaying payment to doctors.

A study showed that an insurance company can make as much as $84,000 in bank interest for each day they delay paying claims. By law an average clean claim (with no errors) should be paid from 14-30 days after a doctor submits the bill. Instead, the average claim is paid anywhere from 30-45 days. Some claims, after multiple appeals, can take up to a year to be paid after the service was given.

6. Insurance companies can ask the doctor for reimbursement for paid claims indefinitely.

A doctor has 120 days to submit a claim for services provided. After that time, he or she may not submit a charge or charge the patient. However, an insurance company can ask for reimbursement from a doctor with no time limit when the company has determined it made an overpayment or paid for services not covered under the contract.

A small but growing number of physicians are opting out of health insurance contracts and instead, providing healthcare on a cash basis. Many of these are also severing their contracts with Medicare and Medicaid. While this gives the physician more freedom, and provides much-needed personal care and pricing transparency for patients, it does beg the question: As an increasing number of physicians go into cash practices, who will care for the millions of Americans who hang on to their insurance cards, or the millions more that ACA-backers are celebrating as they enter Medicaid programs?

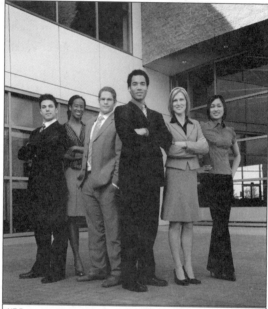

"You can trust us to manage your health and your money. We know what's best for your doctors and you. Just relax."

CHAPTER 22
ACOS COMING RIGHT NOW TO A NEIGHBORHOOD NEAR YOU AND BRINGING BIG DOCTOR RIGHT ALONG

The ACA goes far beyond bundling payments for healthcare, however, as it marches Americans toward total federalization of healthcare for Medicare recipients. Sec. 3022 of the new law requires the establishment of "shared savings program[s]" in the Medicare system. The law states, "The ACO shall be willing to become accountable for the quality, cost, and overall care of the Medicare fee-for-service beneficiaries assigned to it."

An ACO is a large, multi-specialty medical group that includes physicians, surgeons, other medical providers, and facilities. These disparate entities come together ostensibly to provide comprehensive, coordinated care for individuals. ACOs are often associated with providing care for diabetics, individuals with cardiac issues, or those with a combination of chronic medical conditions. In practice, however, ACOs are meant to become the single-shop under which an individual receives medical care.

Remarkably, as ACOs are rolled out, individuals find they are assigned to one simply because their physician signed an ACO contract. The patient, then, is no longer being treated by the physician's clinic, but under the watchful eye of Big Doctor – the ACO. The patient has no say in his or her assignment to an ACO. Government, which controls the reimbursements, has declared it and the patient must obey.

Medicare uses its billing power to force ACOs into compliance with its federal dictates. So when the Congress voted in April 2015 to fix how doctors are reimbursed (HR 2), it may have only served to speed up the federalization process. Under the old law, a complicated calculation based on spending increases and use of medical services required the federal government to adjust payments to physicians. Although, the adjustment is always downward, it has never happened. Instead, each year Congress passed a "Doc Fix" law that maintained or even slightly increased the reimbursements to doctors. The 2015 law Congress passed supposedly fixed the Doc Fix law.

This new "Doc Fix" law will essentially force every physician that cares for Medicare patients to be contracted with an Accountable Care Organization (ACO) within a few years. ACOs are paid lump sums of money to provide care for an individual and the total is split among all the various providers who work for or are contracted with the ACO. The Medicare payment is supposed to cover the entire cost of care, but if some of the money is not spent, it can be retained by the ACO and members will share in the savings. On the other hand, if the ACO spends more on an individual than Medicare pays the ACO to provide care, the ACO will eat the loss. The temptation, then, will be to deny necessary care to an individual to save money for the ACO. The denial of care will grow more tempting once the ACO begins to claw back payments it made to physicians in previous months and years, after determining the physician provided too many services to patients.

As with many features of ObamaCare, patients will not realize what these ACOs mean to them until they face a medical crisis when it may be too late. Refusing care is a tough and dangerous way to save money, but it is the direction in which ObamaCare moves us.

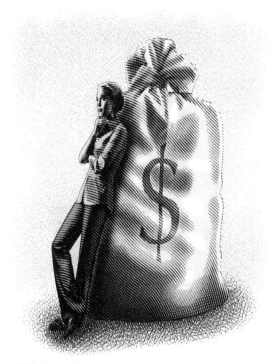

"We have the gold so we write the rules.
Obey the rules and we'll decide how
much to pay you."

Chapter 23
Are High Healthcare Prices Tied To Evidence-Based Medicine?

"Evidence-based healthcare" is one of those undefined, ubiquitous, and too often unquestioned terms so commonly used by healthcare public policy reformers. Everywhere, it seems, people believe evidence-based medicine is key to reforming healthcare. But what exactly is evidence-based medicine?

The U.S. National Center for Clinical Excellence bases the concept of evidence-based medicine on the philosophy, "that as much medical practice as possible ought to be carried out using proven algorithms based on empirically valid evidence from controlled scientific experiments, rather than individual clinical judgment."

Medical practice "evidence" is supposed to result in "practice guidelines" – the theory being that physicians will abide by guidelines based on scientific evidence to direct how they practice medicine instead of their training, experience, insight, intuition, and knowledge of each individual's medical condition. The Affordable Care Act relies heavily on both evidence-based medicine and practice guidelines to set the standards of care for medical treatment and outcomes going forward. Use or disuse of these guidelines can affect whether the physician or hospital receives reimbursement for providing care. Hence, practice guidelines, despite questions about their legitimacy and a paucity of clinical data that they increase the quality of care, will directly affect the quality of and access to care.

Managing healthcare by making payments to Accountable Care Organizations will require the increased use of evidence-based medicine. ACO reimbursements rely on the idea that individual care for any set of medical conditions can be determined through analysis of large numbers in a data set. In this way, asserting that evidence suggests an acceptable protocol of care and tying payment to that protocol will affect how individuals receive care in an ACO.

Medical Master Manager Required

In the first iteration of reform, the U.S. House passed House Bill 3962 in 2009. The bill created a new layer of government bureaucracy that would have inserted itself between the doctor and patient. The bill would have required appointment of a national health commissioner supported by medical task forces to evaluate and decide everything from what medications a physician would be allowed to prescribe for a patient, to what surgery might be approved, to each outcome that would be expected for a particular medical condition. This universal healthcare Czar and the task forces would also have decided whether or not hospitals would be reimbursed for care already provided, based on predetermined outcomes.

(Despite the good news that the medical Czar did not make it into the final ACA bill, we should remain concerned. As the ACA fails to meet its goals, the temptation will to be load it down with more managers, and at some point, the Czar will reemerge.)

For example, if a hospital re-admits a patient within 30 days after discharge, CMS will not reimburse the hospital for care given. Congress' "scientifically-informed wisdom" about this is that the hospital should have provided complete care during the first admission, and not be paid twice if a condition persists. Such a policy, however, does not take into account factors such as how ill a patient may be or the occurrence of a new condition only tangentially related to the original condition. Neither does it account for the patients who fail or refuse to follow the advice of their doctors once they return home from the hospital.

The healthcare Czar would have effectively removed the power of the individual physician and patient to decide what is the best course of treatment. Instead, somewhat like an auto mechanic, the physician would be limited to whatever the manual said regardless of a unique medical condition which the patient presents. When your modern day car develops a thumping sound and is sluggish upon acceleration, your auto repair specialist can plug in an analytical computer program and tell you what is wrong. With this knowledge, the mechanic can apply "evidence-based" repairs and almost always, get it right the first time. If, after you leave the garage, the same conditions exist, you will expect your repairman to fix it at no additional cost. This "evidence-based" repair concept breaks down quickly when applied to humans.

You might feel awful, and even hear sounds in your body that you ascribe to how you feel. Your physician can examine you and "plug in" your conditions to a giant data base from which he or she can find the "evidence-based" practice guidelines for your case. Unlike a car made out of steel and plastic, your body is a literal pool of chemicals and tissue, interacting in unpredictable ways and subject to unpredictable conditions. True enough, a good deal of medical care can be submitted to an algorithmic analysis, and predictions can be made and guidelines offered. But there is no algorithm to anticipate the infinite combination of effects on your body that may occur and cause your sluggishness. That is why physicians practice medicine as an art. If your body breaks down after the hospital releases you, you want to be able to go back and get necessary care, right away without the fear of prohibitive costs that you will be responsible for because Medicare won't pay.

Why should everyday Americans care about a national health Czar prescribing medical care to physicians? The most obvious reason is that the application of evidence-based medicine can potentially limit health choices of both patients and physicians – the limitation of choice could result in reduced quality of care. A reduced quality of care leads to unnecessary pain and suffering, and possibly, premature death.

Stifling alternatives

In HB 3962, the 2009 Congress intended to pressure physicians to deny alternative treatments, and physicians who, based on their best medical knowledge, practiced alternative medicine could have, in some cases, faced criminal charges.

Determining practice guidelines depends on volumes of medical studies, and these studies are expensive. The pharmaceutical industry enjoys providing an ongoing flow of money for studies. Companies without deep pockets, however, would be unable to afford the cost of in-depth studies to critically evaluate the efficacy of alternative treatments. So instead of science proving that alternative treatments are less effective than so-called "evidence-based" treatments it is the lack of funds in many cases that deny researchers the ability to prove the efficacy of those alternative treatments. In short, if alternative treatments are not evaluated based on top-down enforced guidelines of evidence-based medicine, they will never be accepted as a valued treatment option. This is one way in which the pharmaceutical industry can prevent individuals from accessing new, cutting-edge alternative treatments that threaten Big Pharma's profits.

It can also be argued that evidence-based medicine has exponentially increased the cost of healthcare. In theory, the essence of evidence-based medicine is scientific research. In practice, however, it has become more about money. The paucity of money available to pay for some otherwise innovative medical treatments falls against the vast fortunes of the pharmaceutical industry. For example:

- **Many prescription drug trials are not independent**

They are often funded by the same drug companies that stand to gain if their drug is found to be effective in trials and becomes FDA approved.

- **The relationship between medical societies and the pharmaceutical industry raises questions.**

Over the past 10-15 years there has been a change in the parameters of our most common diseases (hypertension, obesity, and high cholesterol). For example, in the past, normal blood pressure was considered to be 120/80, but now it is 115/75. In fact, those with a blood pressure of 120/80 are now considered to be pre-hypertensive and therefore, become eligible for medication. In this case, "evidence-based" medicine is used to justify prescriptions for blood pressure medicine for millions more individuals, and that increases the sales volume for the pharmaceutical companies. If the FDA decided to increase the guidelines for acceptable blood pressure to 130/90, drug sales would plummet and so would pharmaceutical profits.

As a result of "evidence-based medicine," the acceptable body mass index (BMI) number for obesity decreased from 40 to 30 while the parameters for being overweight were expanded from a BMI of 27.8 in 1995 to less than 25 today. No one argues against the fact that Americans, on the whole, are overweight and are less healthy because of it. Yet, it is easy to see how changing the definition of BMI makes it appear more serious than it might otherwise be, and as a result, call for an increase in drug and medical or surgical treatment for obesity.

High cholesterol (LDL) is now considered to be <200 instead of the old parameter of <250. The change in parameters has resulted in both a dramatic increase in the number of people who meet criteria for treatment with prescription drugs and a rise in the price of healthcare. Once again, as a result of this "evidence," physicians are prescribing more statins than ever to control cholesterol.

The question that has yet to be answered is why are Americans less healthy despite taking ever-increasing amounts of prescription medications?

• **There is a tight financial relationship between the pharmaceutical industry and the medical industry.**

The AMA, medical education and the underwriting of medical research has given the pharmaceutical industry a great advantage in the shaping of medical opinion, and given Big Pharma an advantage in evidence-based medicine that favors more consumption of prescription medicine.

• **There is a revolving door between those who work for the FDA and those who have worked in the pharmaceutical industry.**

This cozy relationship raises the importance of Big Pharma and relegates natural/alternative methods to junk science. Inherently, this should make those of us who are critical thinkers question the "experts" that summarily denigrate the health supplement industry and its products that in many cases are in direct competition with the drugs that are manufactured by pharmaceutical companies.

Physicians know that the delivery of healthcare needs to be reformed, improved, and made more affordable and efficient. For a variety of reasons, evidence-based medicine and its practice guidelines will not get us where we need to be. We need a more balanced approach. If we must be forced to live with distant experts evaluating our delivery of healthcare and deciding who will get paid and how much, then at least the same standard should be applied to both alternative and conventional treatments. We would be far better off if each form of treatment is given a level playing field to determine efficacy. This change alone would go a long way toward improving the health of Americans without bankrupting them.

Let's try something new, like promoting prevention and wellness instead of just talking about it. Why not allow doctors and patients the freedom they need to choose how they approach health choices. No one can argue with the fact that a healthier population will lead to a significant decrease in healthcare prices that should reduce overall healthcare spending.

A closing thought. To become a physician, doctors must pass rigorous tests and prove their ability to make sound medical decisions. Science informs them at every step, in addition to their heart and intuition. The more they practice, the more they can practice better medicine. Doctors practice medicine based on the evidence they have learned during their process of education and during clinical application. Modern healthcare gives all physicians who seek it, volumes of evidence upon which to make informed treatment decisions with their patients – without a federal health Czar telling them what to do.

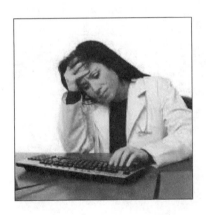

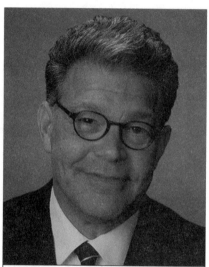

MN Senator Al Franken's 314
vote margin of victory after a
long recount in 2009 gave the
Democrats the 60 votes needed to
pass the PPACA on December 24,
2009.

Chapter 24
Massachusetts Voters took a Stand, but it wasn't enough to Save American Healthcare

During January 2010 Massachusetts voters sent a shot across the bow of Congressional Democrats. The Republican, Scott Brown, won a special election to the United States Senate, thereby reducing the Democratic Senate majority to 59 members. Sen. Ted Kennedy, D-Mass., had succumbed to cancer, and now, the people of Massachusetts had to cast the deciding vote whether or not his legacy healthcare reform bill would be passed. Massachusetts' wise citizens voted against federalizing healthcare when they sent Scott Brown to Washington, DC.

Without their 60 vote majority, the Senate faced unending filibusters that stood the chance of denying them passage of their so-called "Patient Protection and Affordable Care Act." The Senate had passed their first iteration of the bill on Christmas Eve, 2009, not long after Minnesota's Al Franken, the actor and comedian, took his oath of office as the 60th Democrat member, which left the GOP without the ability to stop the vote.

Franken's Election Turned the Tide

Franken's 2008 election, as important as it was in giving the Democrats 60 votes, had been tainted by a dragged out recount in which he finally wrestled victory away from Senator Norm Coleman by 312 votes. Coleman had won the election by 215 votes. The Minnesota election recount, settled in the fall of 2009, left many convinced Franken's party had stolen the election, and once he entered the U.S. Senate, many conservatives felt he would give the Democrats the ability to steal a victory rewriting our healthcare laws.

Then, in 2010, the voters spoke and chose Scott Brown. Brown's January election gave hope to proponents of a more free market approach to healthcare reform. But as it turned out, the Senate used a budget resolution strategy to pass the PPACA on March 23, 2010. The bill the Senate passed had to be amended just 10 days later to resolve differences with the House version. Once Congress passed the new law and President Obama signed it, free market adherents knew they had lost the battle, and wondered if they would eventually lose the war as well.

As an anxious American citizenry watched the Congress fashion ObamaCare, it became more evident by the day that politics drove it, not good healthcare public policy. When it finally passed during March of 2010, thousands of Americans began to come to grips with how Al Franken's election made it possible, followed by the heavy-handed politics of the Democratically-controlled Congress. The politics of the PPACA created the Tea Party movement, an uprising that continued to shake Washington, DC politics through the 2014 election cycle.

Once Congress passed the PPACA (now generally referred to as the Affordable Care Act) it became clear that "healthcare reform" had nothing to do with delivering quality medical care to the American people.

The ACA is a Wolf in Sheep's Clothing

The idea of universal insurance (health plan) coverage, with protection against insurance company wrongs (e g , denying patients for pre-existing conditions and limiting the insurance company's ability to deny coverage when it is needed) served as the sheep's clothing that cloaked the true nature of the ACA – designed to destroy our healthcare system as we knew it. The more we learn about the ACA, in fact, the more we have discovered that it has the potential to make us sicker by limiting our access to necessary treatment, and limiting our choice of physicians while making us pay more for the privilege.

The 2010 U.S. Senate election of Scott Brown in Massachusetts served as a stand against those in the government who are bent on telling us that they know what is best for us. Yet the Congressional Democrats simply used a procedural strategy to thwart the will of the people.

I have been repeatedly astonished by the complete contempt in which those in power hold the American people. A majority of

Americans in 2010 believed the ACA took us in the wrong direction. The vote in Massachusetts should have made the peoples' opposition clear. Yet we saw that Congress ignored the majority, believing that someday, Americans would see their way and congratulate the Democrats with everlasting Congressional majorities. I believe President Obama felt that Americans would nearly canonize him once the bill passed and its enforcement began.

Speaker of the House Nancy Pelosi, D-CA, will forever be saddled with her quote, "We have to pass the bill to find out what is in the bill." An astute physician, in commenting on Pelosi's quote added, "That's the definition of a stool sample." What we've learned about the ACA fits the physician's observation well.
We learned we were saddled with:

- An enormous government bureaucracy run by a universal healthcare Czar in the person of the Secretary of Health and Human Services that will ultimately decide what will be covered. The Secretary could be the arbiter about whether or not a patient receives needed medical care, like a hip replacement or gene therapy.

- A commission appointed by the president that will decide what treatments will be allowed for what diseases (the commission is mandated to have only one physician).

- A government-run committee driven by evidence-based medicine that will decide clinical outcomes. If the expected outcome is not achieved then the provider will not be paid.

- A government able to decide whether a hospital will be paid for services rendered. For example, if a patient is re-admitted to a hospital in a shorter time than the government deems appropriate, then the hospital will not be paid. It does not take into account how ill the patient may be.

Although Scott Brown's election should have been seen as a win for opponents of Washington, DC-controlled healthcare reform, we witnessed the sheer hypocrisy of the Democrats as they voted to pass this assault on liberty and common sense. Passing the ACA only added to America's frustration over other incidences in which Congress pushed through unpopular legislation – does TARP ring a bell?

The ACA passed without a single Republican vote, because Democrats wanted to own the new law. Their arrogance and disregard for the voters' wishes sent many of them packing after the 2010 election. By 2014, voters had said "enough" and gave majorities to the Republicans in both the U.S. House and Senate.

I believe that had President Obama been on the ballot in 2014, voters would have sent him packing as well. He, along with Congressional Democrats, should have listened to the Massachusetts voters in 2010.

The challenge for voters after 2014 is to hold the new GOP House and Senate majority's feet to the fire, and use all means to persuade President Obama to bend his stubborn will to allow reform of his ill-named Affordable Care Act. Certainly, the roll out of the federal and state health insurance exchanges should be enough to convince the GOP it must do something, despite the president's stubbornness.

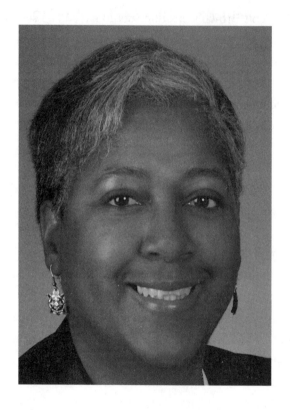

CHAPTER 25
A PRACTICING PHYSICIAN'S
PRESCRIPTION FOR A HEALTHCARE FIX

For all of the desperate attempts at distraction, demonization and outright lies about ObamaCare, the truth remains: Enrolling in a health plan is not the same as gaining access to quality healthcare.

The healthcare finance system, including public and private health plans, is in trouble. If healthcare reform "experts" had bothered to ask independent private physicians about problems with getting paid for providing healthcare services, perhaps the reformers would have found solutions that work. Instead, the staff and consultants that put the ACA together drew knowledge from and were convinced by the staff and consultants who worked for powerful interest groups.

Reformers could have asked, why are an increasing number of physicians refusing to take Medicare or Medicaid patients? Why are physicians and surgeons opting out of accepting any type of health insurance payments? Why are more physicians moving toward a cash-only practice, altogether freed from the third party reimbursement system? If the reformers had found answers to these questions, then they may have searched for improvements in how to link up individuals with these cash-practice doctors. It didn't happen because they never asked physicians, and if they had asked, the AMA, PhARMa, AHIP, AARP, NAHU, NAIFA, Families Forever, and a long list of other advocacy groups they would have shouted them down.

Had the reformers asked, physicians would have explained that the game is rigged. It has become harder for doctors to offer, and patients to access quality affordable healthcare. As a result of the reformers' failure to talk with private physicians, ObamaCare expanded and empowered the wrong people. Instead of strengthening the patient-physician relationship, ObamaCare empowered those who control the most expensive aspects of our healthcare system – huge medical provider systems, insurance companies, pharmaceutical companies, and thousands of new MediCrats.[30] The reformers have thereby doomed Americans to paying more for health insurance and paying more taxes, while increasingly facing rationed healthcare.

In what many believe to be candor but which is, in reality, an expression of chutzpah, the Obama White House now tells us that we spent 27.5 percent of our income taxes on healthcare.[30] This ratio is a 20 percent increase in just two years between 2012 and 2014, and shows the direction in which our health expenditures are

---

[30] Weber, R. MediCrats: Medical Bureaucrats that Rule your Health Care. Alethos Press. St. Paul, MN. 2013. "A health care bean counter working for a government or regulatory agency, a large health plan/insurance company, or medical provider whose primary task is to control the health of a nation's residents and the payment systems allowed to cover health services." P 1.

[31] Your 2014 Taxpayer Receipt. The White House. Retrieved on 4/16/2015. https://www.whitehouse.gov/2014-taxreceipt

going, thanks to the ACA. Health expenditures, as a part of the federal budget, is now the single largest category of spending. Based on what we have seen since the ACA kicked in, this will grow each year, choking out other federal programs; that is, until the federal government reverses course and, in the name of frugality, begins to order reductions in spending. Federal reductions means reduced medical services for everyone.

Now that Congress has passed the ACA, the proponents of ObamaCare like Ezekiel Emanuel (the architect of The Complete Lives System) and columnist/economist Paul Krugman are finally admitting the truth. ObamaCare's authors intended to control our healthcare system by centralizing power in the federal government. To control costs, ObamaCare empowers a vast bureaucracy funded by higher taxes whose purpose is to ration healthcare (i.e., death panels). One result is that 30 million people who were previously uninsured will be exchanged for those who had insurance but were not dependent on government handouts to pay for it.

ObamaCare transfers wealth from the young and the middle class to the government and its corporate friends. More than the money, however, as an astute individual commented – it is actually a transfer of health. Americans are losing their freedom to choose their doctor, and their freedom to choose how they prefer to treat their illness. For example, under ObamaCare, people can no longer use their Health Savings Account (HSA) to buy natural remedies such as vitamins and supplements. Concerning medicines, the new law limits HSAs to the purchase of brand name or generic prescription drugs.

Looking forward, it seems inevitable that more restrictions and mandates must follow those already in place. How long will it be, for instance, before government "experts" will mandate that we must take vaccines, and if we refuse, be placed on psychiatric medication against our will?

The nature of a collectivist system such as that created by ObamaCare, is that administrative cost soars, and the result is a loss of individual freedom. To better manage cost, federal officials will use private medical data accessed through the national electronic medical record database from which they will devise an algorithm and claim it can predict success of medical intervention.

Robert Geist, MD, is a retired urologist in Minnesota. In an email message related to the 2015 passage of the so-called "Doc Fix," Geist reached back to a prediction he made when Health Maintenance Organizations (HMOs) first arrived on the scene. It is chilling to think that Geist might have nailed down so long ago what will eventually have to happen going forward.

> Which bring to mind the next nasty gimmick possible. 40 years ago I predicted that the HMOs would sell only patient compliant contracts. For instance if the patient missed 50% of prenatal visits, the mother was responsible for 50% of the bill. If the body fat index did not decrease as ordered, financial penalties or even loss of insurance would ensue. If an ultrasound showed any deformity and an abortion was refused, the patient paid all maternity costs... The HMO lobby

brought up patient compliance contracts to Congress in about 1980 and there was a Minnesota push around the same time. Even our liberal friends recoiled at the time and these efforts went no place.

I expect some sort of compliance will be part of future cartel insurance contracts. You can probably think of many examples of what will be penalized. Not taking medications is the first that comes to mind. I think all inhibitions regarding MBA-ACO-HMO diktats are now off the shelf. Any "final solution" is possible when patients and doctor cost centers need to be threatened and when "necessary," given the maximum financial penalties. How about refusing an assisted suicide or pulling the plug on really sick or just old "crumbly" people? So who is next, the "unproductive?"[32]

My Solutions To Reform The Current System

So much good could have been done if reformers had asked physicians for solutions, instead of creating a vast new bureaucracy. These are some simple solutions I would recommend if I were asked:

- **Change the tax code to allow private physicians to write off bad debt.**

Allow physicians to write off delinquent patient bills as bad debt.

[32] Geist, R., MD. (2015) In email addressed to members of the Minnesota Physician-Patient Alliance. 4/16/2015. St Paul, MN. Retrieved on 4/16/2015.

This would alleviate the need to send the patient to collections. It would reduce the number of bankruptcies resulting from health-care costs. It would also encourage more charitable medical care because physicians could afford to offer it.

- ## Change medical malpractice laws through tort reform

Require patients and the attorneys that represent them who file frivolous malpractice lawsuits to pay all court costs. Establish monetary caps on punitive damage awards paid to patients. Encourage doctors to provide free care by giving them a discount on their malpractice insurance or waiving it if they provide a specified level of free care per year.

- ## Allow Medicare and Medicaid access to cheaper drugs from other countries

Allow importation of FDA-approved drugs from foreign countries for use by Medicare and Medicaid patients. Provide access to these drugs for all government employees that receive health insurance as an employee benefit.

- ## Reform EMTALA - The Emergency Medical Treatment and Active Labor Act

This is an unfunded congressional mandate passed in 1986 that requires hospital emergency rooms to treat all patients regardless of their ability to pay. Hospitals, forced to accept these non-paying patients, pass along these costs to patients who are able to pay.

Instead: Require that patients who present to the emergency room be triaged and treated for real emergencies only, and not problems that are best treated in an outpatient office, clinic, or urgent care setting, e.g., common cold or ear-wax removal. Then free the hospitals from any further legal requirement to offer treatment.

- **Require insurance companies to honor the pre-certification process**

Require that if an insurance company pre-certifies (approves) a procedure then they have to pay for it. They cannot deny it after the fact and leave the patient on the hook for paying the bill.

- **Separate the triumvirate of the pharmacies, insurance companies (health plans) and pharmacy benefit management companies (PBMs)**

The collusion between insurance companies, pharmacies, and PBMs serves to keep prescription medication cost higher than necessary, and limits the competition among drug manufacturers that is necessary to reduce the cost of medicine.

- **Refuse to mandate, as a matter of licensure, that physicians must accept Medicare, Medicaid or ObamaCare health insurance plans**

The best way to encourage physicians to leave the practice of medicine and find new professions is to force them to accept Medicaid, Medicare, and ObamaCare insured patients. Let this remain voluntary, and allow the marketplace to work it out. Put this into statute to make it harder for a future president to declare it by an executive order.

- **Reform medical insurance so that funds paid for medical expenses that did not reach the deductible amounts would rollover to the next year so that they could be used as a credit that would limit out-of-pocket expenses for patients.**

Under this idea, if a patient had a $2,500 deductible, but only spent $500 in a year, they would have a credit of $2,000 that would rollover to the next year. She/he would then only have to pay a maximum of $2,000 dollars under the deductible before the insurance would pay for additional covered medical expense. After the patient has paid up to the deductible, the following year the deductible would reset to $2,500.

CHAPTER 26
WHAT THE KING V BURWELL DECISION MEANS FOR DOCTORS AND PATIENTS

While reading the June 25, 2015 Supreme Court decision in <u>King v. Burwell</u>, I realized that the ruling did not surprise me. It fits the pattern that has developed over the last several years. The Court has made it clear – when it comes to the Affordable Care Act, the letter of the law is not important.

We first saw this in the 2012 decision <u>NFIB v. Sibelius</u>. The Court upheld the ACA by saying the individual mandate wasn't a mandate, but a tax. The Court did this to avoid declaring the mandate as an abrogation of the Commerce Clause. The <u>NFIB</u> case turned syntax and definitions on their head. With King the Court has outdone itself. The Court has massaged the meaning of subsidies that apply only to state run exchanges, as the law clearly states, to apply to all government exchanges, to everyone.

The Court ignores the most important fact that patients will continue to find access to healthcare limited by rising out-of-pocket expenses in the form of rising deductibles, co-insurance, and premiums that are expected to continue to spike much higher.

As a result, we can continue to look forward to patients using emergency rooms as primary care centers because they can't afford to see a physician. We will see more independent physicians closing their practices or becoming hospital employees, further exacerbating the doctor shortage. The ruling does nothing to change the reality that having health insurance in the age of ObamaCare does not equal access to quality healthcare.

Finally, the winners have been rewarded. When the stock value of health related companies such as corporate hospitals rise on the news of the decision, doctors and patients should take notice. The insurance companies and hospitals have clearly figured out that business as usual can continue. In fact, it will become business as usual on steroids.

Insurance companies will be empowered to further limit their physician panels, they will continue to decrease the medications that they will cover, they will continue to decrease what they cover as medically unnecessary and experimental in order to limit access to physician directed care while they increase their premiums increasing their profits in the bargain. Hospitals will continue to get larger taking over the market and setting prices without pressure from honest competition from independent physicians, ambulatory surgery centers, labs and radiology centers that would encourage cost control.

The King v. Burwell decision has answered the question of who stands to gain in the age of Obamacare. Justice Roberts in his opinion said it best "Congress passed the Affordable Care Act to improve health insurance markets, not to destroy them." With this decision, medical insurance companies, hospitals and other pieces of the corporate healthcare delivery system now have the scale clearly tipped in their favor at the expense of doctors and their patients – mission accomplished.

Chapter 27
This Doctor's Rx for
Healthcare Reform

Think about it. If the government's primary purpose in passing the ACA really was to enroll 30 million uninsured people into a health plan, all the law needed to do was expand Medicaid. This would be far more efficient and less costly than blowing up the private insurance market. The fact is that the ACA authors meant to do much more; to federalize the practice of and payment for healthcare.

The most effective and efficient healthcare reform, however, would be to empower independent doctors instead of creating schemes that build massive provider systems based in the hospitals, paid for by Big Insurance, and highly influenced by Big Pharma. We can have real, effective healthcare reform that gives Americans access to quality, affordable healthcare. It all starts in the physician's exam room, not in a Washington, D.C. bureaucrat's office.

I have been in medical practice more than 15 years. Over the past several years I have written extensively about both the intended and the unintended consequences of federal healthcare reform from a physician's perspective.

My motive in writing about healthcare is simple. As a physician I have unique knowledge about how the healthcare system works. I have witnessed firsthand the erosion and breakdown of the patient-doctor relationship, which is tragic as it is the fundamental foundation of medicine.

As a doctor I am, by definition, a patient advocate. As with a medical diagnosis that will affect my patient's life going forward, I am compelled to educate and inform people about what to expect over the coming months and years regarding their healthcare choices resulting from federal healthcare reform.

I started my journey to affect change in healthcare as an idealistic optimist who believed that my voice could be heard. That belief took me to Washington, D.C., to meet with my Congressmen where I learned a hard lesson. I found in the halls of Congress that the political status quo and the power of special interests were more important to lawmakers than doing what is best for patients. It exacerbated my frustration as I watched politics play an increasing role in how I was told to deliver medical care to my patients.

It has been equally frustrating to listen to pundits talk about the delivery of medical care. Most pundits know absolutely nothing about what it takes to keep a practice open and to provide excellent care to patients. I found myself shaking my head in disbelief as I heard a pundit opine about the role of the doctor when I knew the pundit never had to make a payroll or pay for malpractice insurance, or had navigated the insurance maze to make sure my patient was able to receive the care they needed. How many reporters have had to fight increasingly more losing battles with insurance companies and the government for the chance to treat a patient as they were trained to do? Where do these reporters get the authority to dictate to doctors the course of conversations on healthcare reform?

Finally, I came full circle. I decided to quit complaining about the problem and, instead, do something to be part of the solution. Each of us needs to make this decision, in a wide array of instances.

- Instead of complaining about how we are losing jobs to other countries, why don't we just pay a little more to buy from those who make things here in the USA?

- Instead of complaining about illegal immigration, why don't we make the choice to trade and do business with companies that can document that they follow the rule of law and hire documented workers?

In the United States we get what we pay for. Each of has to make a choice about what to buy and from whom. Our purchasing decisions will have far more impact than whom we choose to serve in Congress. Whoever controls the purse strings controls the power. With that in mind, the future stability of the American healthcare system rests on removing the middlemen that drive up the cost of care, and limit its practice – the government and commercial insurance companies. The answer lies in healthcare consumerism where price transparency and competition between healthcare professionals reign.

Many examples of free market medicine are found across the country. Surgical services delivered by independent surgery centers (e.g., www.surgerycenterok.com); high quality urgent care centers run by ER board certified physicians that offer medical services for a flat rate (e.g., www.atlantaurgentcare.com); direct pay practices with a subscription that will deliver comprehensive care including discount prescriptions and labs for a flat monthly fee (e.g., www.atlasmd/wichita/); practices that offer a sliding scale for patients who will pay cash each time they see a doctor, and which works with the individual patient's budget (e.g. www.aapsonline.org) ; practices which barter (e.g., www.southern barterclub.com); medical cost sharing (which is allowed under Obamacare) to cover necessary medical care, dental care, prescriptions, holistic care, chiropractic care, and catastrophic care (e.g., www.libertyoncall.org); and supplemental policies such as Aflac (e.g., www.aflac.com) paired with comprehensive coverage for catastrophic medical conditions such as cancer and heart disease, as well as ICU coverage. Each of these strategies put the power back with the doctor and the patient and removes the bureaucracy that fuels prohibitive healthcare costs. If unleashed from government and insurance company overseers, the variety of types of practices and how to pay for services would erupt – innovation would happen.

I have incorporated the subscription, sliding scale, and barter models as strategies in my medical practice. I have chosen to use Liberty HealthShare and Aflac for myself and my employees to opt out of the broken healthcare system. My choices have given me back my power as a physician, and instead of thinking of leaving medicine, I have rediscovered the joy of being a physician. I once again practice medicine with the Hippocratic Oath as the foundation without duress. It is empowering to know that I have the tools to help myself and I no longer feel forced to sit back and hope that the Government will help me.

When Congress passed the Patient Protection and Affordable Care Act, it made it plain that politicians have a different plan for America than we doctors do. You only have to look to the increased stock value of the pharmaceutical and insurance companies to know who the winners were in the PPACA debate.

Many politicians made their choice by voting for ObamaCare, and their votes were followed by governors and state legislators across the country. We know where they stand, and recent elections show that the voters do, too, and have thrown many of them out of office. We need to continue this trend, and as physicians, help to inform our patients.

We doctors, however, cannot wait for politicians to get the message. We already know the message – now we must share it with our patients and the public.

My Rx for healthcare reform is for doctors to do what we do best; diagnose the problem and recommend a therapy. But in the case of reforming healthcare, we have to do more than advise our patients what to do; we have to directly confront the political forces and economic interests that undermine our patients and our profession by withdrawing our consent. When we once again value ourselves as healers, our patients will join with us and together we can elevate the standard of care bringing individuality, empathy and humanity back to medicine. As necessary, physicians need to change the way we do business and in some cases, it means we stop playing the game neither we nor our patients can win.

It is in our hands to cure our healthcare system.

About Elaina George, MD, and How to Contact Her

Elaina George, MD is a Board Certified Otolaryngologist. She graduated from Princeton University with a degree in Biology. She received her Master's degree in Medical Microbiology from Long Island University, and received her medical degree from Mount Sinai School of Medicine in New York. Dr George completed her residency at 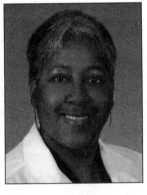 Manhattan, Eye Ear & Throat Hospital. Her training included general surgery at Lenox Hill Hospital, pediatric ENT at The NY-Presbyterian Hospital, and head and neck oncology at Memorial Sloan-Kettering Cancer Center. She has published in several scientific journals and presented her research at national meetings.

Dr. George is in solo practice at the Peachtree Ear, Nose & Throat Center, in Atlanta, Georgia. – http://www.peachtreeentcenter.com Dr. George blogs at http://drelainageorge.com.

As a solo practitioner in private practice, Dr. George is also a small business owner, which offers her a unique perspective on the problems of health care delivery, the true costs of healthcare, and viable solutions.

Dr George received the Patients' Choice Award in 2008 and 2009. She was recently honored with membership in "The Leading Physicians of the World" and "Who's Who Top Doctors, Honors Edition."

Dr George's interest in the politics of healthcare and the reform effort have led her to become both a powerful voice for the practicing physician and an advocate for the patient.

She serves on the advisory council of Project 21 black leadership network, an initiative of The National Center for Public Policy Research. She is a contributor to a wide variety of websites including BigGovernment.com, Newmediajournal.us, and Amy Ridenour's National Center Blog. Dr George has been a recurring guest discussing a wide range of medical topics on Your World with Neil Cavuto, and Newsmax, and she has appeared on Frances & Friends to discuss the consequences of Obamacare with a worldwide audience of over 500 million people.

Dr. George has also been a medical expert on a range of other radio and TV shows including The Barry Farber Show, The Chuck Wilder Show, and Butler on Business. Dr George hosts her own show, *Medicine On Call* on America's Web Radio and LibertyTalk.fm, a weekly talk show that explores health issues and the politics of medicine.

She is also a keynote speaker offered through CSL Entertainment and American Entertainment International.

To contact Dr. George as a speaker or for media inquiries contact 404-840-0415 or email <u>dynomuse@aol.com</u>.

To Contact the Publisher:

Alethos Press
1535 Barclay Street, Ste B-1
St Paul MN 55106-1405
651.340.1911

<u>http://www.alethospress.com</u>

SOME OF DR. GEORGE'S FAVORITE RESOURCES

Georgia

North Atlanta Urgent Care (www.atlantaurgentcare.com) An urgent care center run by ER board certified physicians that charges a flat fee that covers care.

Highland Urgent Care (www.hucfm.com) A full service urgent care clinic that offers comprehensive primary care services. The urgent care center posts prices for services and the primary care clinic has a subscription based plan and a comprehensive holistic/metabolic complimentary practice.

Peachtree Ear, Nose & Throat Center ENT
www.peachtreeentcenter.com

ENT services specializing in minimally invasive sinus and nasal surgery including balloon sinus dilation, septoplasty. Allergy testing and treatment with sublingual immunotherapy and general/holistic ENT. Offers subscription a based plan, direct pay sliding scale, or barter.

Women for Women - Holistic Gynecology –
www.wmn4wmn.com - Felicia Dawson, MD. A practice that
specializes in holistic gynecology

Holistic Gynecology, Inc.
www.holisticgynecology.com - Juaquita D. Callaway, MD. A
practice that specializes in holistic gynecology and fertility.

Florida

Epiphany Health
www.prime-health.us – A direct primary care practice that specializes in affordable individualized patient care. "Concierge care
for the little guy."

Kansas

Atlas MD – www.atlas/wichita – A flagship direct pay practice
that offers pharmacy services and comprehensive primary care
services for the whole family for one low monthly subscription
fee.

New Jersey

Zarephath – www.zhcenter.org – A health center in Somerset, NJ
that provides free healthcare to those who are poor or uninsured.
It is staffed by volunteer physicians.

Oklahoma

The Surgery Center of Oklahoma – www.surgerycenterok.com – A multispecialty independent surgery center that posts its prices online – prices include all costs associated with the procedure.

National

Aflac – www.Aflac.com/steve_money Policies that pay for high healthcare costs such as cancer diagnosis, MI, stroke and hospitalization. A great adjunct to high deductible policies and medical cost sharing plans (see Liberty HealthShare)

American Association of Physicians and Surgeons – www.aapsonline.org – A professional organization that represents independent physician nationwide. It is a resource for both doctors and patients.

Citizen's Council For Health Freedom – www.cchfreedom.org Twila Brase, former ER Nurse, is the President & Co-founder of Citizens' Council for Health Freedom. Protecting the mission of medicine from the business of healthcare. An important resource which examines rarely discussed issues that affect patients, especially patient privacy

Doctors 4 Patient Care – https://d4pcfoundation.org – An advocacy organization that represents doctors and patients and advocates for the doctor patient relationship

Liberty HealthShare – www.libertyoncall.org – A medical cost sharing company, allowed under ObamaCare (no fines) that covers individuals and families nationwide providing affordable comprehensive coverage for medical, pharmacy, dental, surgical, holistic, chiropractic, and hospital care for a fraction of what private insurance costs. No doctor or hospital panels - open access to see any MD or go to any hospital.

Medibid – www.medibid.com – A service that gives the patient to bid for medical and surgical services from doctors nationwide.

Alethos Press – www.alethospress.com – Publisher, offering truth in narrative.

www.infowars.life – Excellent high quality supplements

www.youngevity.com – Excellent high quality supplements

www.naturalnews.com – Excellent source for health information

Books

Sean Parnell – *The Self Pay Patient: Affordable Health Care Choices in the Age of ObamaCare.* www.theselfpaypatient.com Practical information on how to navigate the healthcare system if you have no insurance or if you have a high deductible insurance policy. Also provides practical advice on how to negotiate a reduced hospital bill for pennies on the dollar.